Having a Cesarean Baby

RICHARD HAUSKNECHT, M.D. is Associate Clinical Professor of Obstetrics and Gynecology at Mount Sinai School of Medicine in New York City and Associate Attending Obstetrician at Mount Sinai Hospital. He also has a private practice in New York City.

JOAN RATTNER HEILMAN is a medical writer and mother of three children. She is the co-author of several books including *The Complete Book of Midwifery*, with Barbara Brennan, C.N.M.

⌘ Having a ⌘ Cesarean Baby

NEWLY REVISED

Richard Hausknecht, M.D.
Joan Rattner Heilman

E.P. DUTTON, / NEW YORK

PHOTOGRAPHS BY ABIGAIL HEYMAN

Published in the United States by E. P. Dutton,
2 Park Avenue, New York, N.Y. 10016

LIBRARY OF CONGRESS CATALOG CARD NUMBER: 82-72516

ISBN: 0-525-93266-6

10 9 8 7 6 5 4 3

Second Edition

Contents

Some Personal Thoughts

There are many personal reasons for writing a book for cesarean parents. First of all, while there are a great number of books on childbirth, none of them has devoted more than a few paragraphs to cesarean birth. There has been no way for parents to inform themselves about having a baby in this alternate way.

But our motives also include the idea that perhaps we can have some small influence on the way obstetrics is practiced in the United States today. As an obstetrician and gynecologist, specializing in high-risk pregnancies and associated with one of the most respected medical centers in the world, I feel that the quality of obstetrical care in this country is not as good as it could and should be, especially when a cesarean birth is necessary. Even where technical skill is satisfactory, the *emotional* aspects of the birthing process are usually ignored.

People in the hands of the medical establishment have a right to know what is happening to them and why it is happening. These are their bodies and their lives, and they have the right to participate in decisions involving them. Changes in the patterns of medical care almost always originate in pressure from the consumers—the patients—and this is a major reason for providing them with facts.

The trend in this country is toward a whole new way of having babies—not only when they arrive in the usual way through the birth canal, but also when they are delivered in a cesarean birth. The trend is toward a dignified, shared, informed, family-oriented childbirth; it recognizes that having a baby is an intensely emotional experience and should be a happy and joyous occasion. For cesarean parents, the new trend is only just beginning. Because the birth experience is literally and entirely taken out of their control and the baby is delivered by a team of professionals in a surgical procedure, they have been left behind and left out, and the birth of their baby has often been treated almost as a side effect of an abdominal operation.

Because so many new parents have been bitterly disappointed by missing out on what they thought was going to be a peak experience in their lives, because they have felt they were casually or even cruelly treated, and because they have begun to speak out individually and collectively as consumers, cesarean parents are finally joining other parents in seeking and finding a positive birth experience.

So this book is written in the hope that it will add fuel to the flickering fire of change that is beginning in obstetrics. It is also a rather plaintive cry for a change in the academic training programs in the medical schools where young men and women are learning to become obstetricians and gynecologists. These men and women are taught medical expertise—obviously of enormous importance—but they are taught little or nothing about the human aspects of childbirth: prepared childbirth, breastfeeding, parent-infant bonding, husband participation, the emotional components of the birthing experience, communication, compassion. All of these things are learned, if indeed they are learned at all, on the job.

There is a great disparity in the availability of first-class medical care in this country. In some institutions and even areas, superb technical care is available to everyone. In others, the general level is poor, and in some, only those with adequate incomes receive the best treatment. Often there are too many hospitals trying to match the facilities of neighboring institutions, with substandard results. And obstetrics has become so specialized, practiced by a very limited number of physicians aided by a battery of electronic gadgetry, that childbirth has tended to be depersonalized.

People deserve individualized medical care, understanding, and support—probably most importantly when they are having a baby because so many lives and relationships are involved. They deserve to be made *partners with the doctor,* even when the birth will be cesarean and requires surgery. They deserve explanations, information, and reassurance about all those things which to us as physicians seem so obvious and necessary but which can be so threatening to lay people. They are entitled to a birth experience that gives them as much pleasure and as little difficulty as we can help them to have.

This book, we hope, will be a step toward helping both the medical establishment and new parents understand that *cesarean births can be just as meaningful and joyful as other methods of childbirth.* A cesarean birth is not merely a surgical procedure; essentially it is the birth of a new life, and the manner in which that new life is greeted can affect the relationship between parents and child far into the future.

It is time that cesarean parents received the attention, understanding, support, and information they need to help them anticipate their birth experience with enthusiasm and look back on it with joy.

RICHARD HAUSKNECHT, M.D.
New York City

Having a Cesarean Baby

1

So You Are Having a Cesarean Baby

If you are reading this book, you are probably about to have a cesarean birth, or you have just had one. And you are not at all unusual. One out of every five babies born in the United States today arrives by this route. That means about 500,000 a year, and many more than ever before in history.

Twenty-five years ago, a hospital with a cesarean section rate of more than 5 percent (one in twenty) was considered to be doing a poor job of obstetrics. But today it is considered inappropriate, and probably dangerous, if a major hospital's rate falls below about 12 percent (about one in eight). In some large urban medical centers, as many as a quarter of the infants come into the world by cesarean.

A cesarean birth is the birth of your baby through incisions in your abdominal and uterine walls. It is also called an abdominal birth. Though it obviously requires a surgical operation, it is the birth of a child, the start of a new family unit, and one of the most significant events in your life. It can be just as happy, fulfilling, and satisfying as any other delivery if you know *why* and *how* it is happening, and if you understand that its purpose is to deliver a normal healthy baby that might have had a difficult or even impossible time being born in the traditional way. It is not abnormal, it is simply an alternate method of birth for sixteen out of every 100 babies born in this country today.

Most women know surprisingly little about cesarean birth, even after they have had one. But with the dramatic increase in the numbers of babies born this way, they are beginning to educate and prepare themselves so they can be more relaxed, feel more in control of their bodies and their emotions, and play a significant role in some of the decision-making concerning themselves and their babies.

This book is intended to help you, a prospective cesarean parent, do that—to answer the questions you have about cesarean birth; to allay your fears and apprehensions; to explain clearly the procedures, causes, possible effects, and common psychological responses; and to help you make your baby's birth a good experience. If you have already had an abdominal birth, our intention is to help you understand just what it was that happened, and why—and to let you know that your physical and emotional responses to a cesarean birth are both common and normal.

WHY SO MANY CESAREAN BIRTHS TODAY?

No one really knows just how a cesarean section got its name, but it seems certain that it did not come about because Julius Caesar was born this way. In Caesar's day, women never survived abdominal births, and it is known that Caesar's mother lived for many years after he arrived. One theory holds that there was a Roman law known as *lex caesarea* that ordered that women who died in the last few weeks of their pregnancies were to be "sectioned" so that their child could be buried separately. Another possibility is that the word *cesarean* derives from the Latin verb *caedere*, "to cut."

Until modern times, cesarean births were rarely, if ever, successful in saving the lives of either mothers or babies. As a result, throughout history they were used only in the most desperate situations—usually in an attempt to salvage the baby of a dying mother. As surgical methods improved, abdominal birth became an alternate method of last resort, when a childbirth became so threatening that there was nothing else to do.

But today, because cesarean delivery has become one of the safest of major operations, doctors use it not only when life or health is threatened, but also as a precautionary measure—a way to prevent problems that may arise and to avoid potential trouble. It is so safe and easy, in fact, that it may occasionally be chosen when it is not really needed.

Cesarean birth became so safe because of many scientific advances. Marked improvements in surgical anesthesia, the discovery of antibiotics, improved surgical techniques, and the availability of blood transfusions all combined to bring about a dramatic drop in maternal mortality (down to less than 0.01 percent nationwide) and fetal mortality, as well as in damaged babies (newborn morbidity), and a significant rise in the number of cesarean births. In many hospitals, the number of cesarean births has doubled, sometimes even tripled, in the last ten years.

Other factors have played an important role in increasing the numbers of abdominal deliveries. There has been an almost universal decision among obstetricians to deliver the majority of first breech babies by cesarean because the risks are lower. (A breech baby is any baby delivered buttocks or feet first.) Also, women with diseases such as diabetes and chronic hypertension that once precluded successful pregnancy can now, with medical help, become pregnant and produce children. Some of these babies are delivered surgically because in this way the perhaps-fragile fetuses are protected from the traumas they might encounter during a normal labor.

Concern for the well-being and health of the fetus and newborn baby has grown in recent years as well. Because fewer babies are being born and family size is diminishing, every baby today is considered to be at a premium. If, in a particular case, a cesarean birth is more likely to produce a healthy baby, it will be the method that is chosen.

Another major factor responsible for the large increase in cesarean births is the fetal monitor. The use of electronic fetal-heart-rate monitoring to detect unborn babies who may be in trouble has rapidly become a standard practice throughout the United States, and several studies have indicated that when a hospital begins to use the monitors, there is a sharp and sudden rise in its cesarean section rate.

There has been considerable controversy about the validity and interpretation of the monitor findings, and allegations that many babies are making their way into the world via totally unnecessary surgery. Though the monitors have certainly saved many infants from damage or even death by pinpointing more accurately than could have been done before which babies seemed to be in danger during labor, it is also true that some cesareans are inappropriate.

Interpreting the data revealed by the monitors isn't always easy, and medical personnel are not always as sophisticated as their machines. In some rare cases, monitors can malfunction. And there is a tendency, if any of the information seems at all out of the ordinary, to rush to the operating room. Partly, this tendency can be explained by the attitudes "Better safe than sorry" and "Why *not* do a cesarean since it's so easy?"

At the root of a great many surgical deliveries is the very real threat of malpractice suits. Many physicians have become so intimidated by the possibility of lawsuits that they often take no chances of being accused—perhaps as many as eighteen years later—of not having done everything they could have, even though the reasons for performing a cesarean may have been quite unclear. So the method is often used to prevent a problem that *may* arise.

Certainly in the case of breech deliveries, the threat of malpractice has been responsible for the almost universal delivery of breeches in the first pregnancy by cesarean, especially because doctors now hesitate to use forceps for the same reason. Clearly, the fear of malpractice suits is in the mind of all obstetricians, the most sued group of doctors in the United States.

The vast majority of cesarean births, however, occur as the result of careful and concerned professional medical judgment. The object is to deliver a healthy baby, undamaged by the tribulations of a difficult and complicated vaginal birth.

WHEN YOU NEED A CESAREAN

Let's face it, few women would *choose* to have a cesarean birth (except in Brazil, where it has become fashionable and accounts for 60 percent of the private deliveries), even though it may be greeted with relief after many hours of a difficult labor. A major abdominal operation is nobody's idea of heaven. There are physical discomforts, restrictions on your mobility and your strength, and the inevitable period of recovery.

However, that doesn't mean it cannot be a happy and emotionally gratifying experience. With preparation, you can manage, as many cesarean mothers do, to get through the physical discomforts without too much difficulty and to focus on the main event: the birth of your baby.

If you have advance notice that you are going to be a cesarean mother or that the possibility exists for you (and to tell the truth, it exists for every pregnant woman), you must set about educating yourself—finding out everything you can in order to know what to expect, and how best to cope with it, and to know your options and your rights.

By reading this book and any other literature you can

find; communicating closely with your obstetrician; visiting the hospital where you will have the baby, and taking a look at the delivery or operating room; speaking, if you can arrange it, with the anesthesiologist; taking a prepared-childbirth course specifically designed for cesarean parents or a class that includes at least a session or two on cesarean birth (if your class doesn't, ask for it); joining a cesarean parents support group (there are more and more forming each year around the country) where you can hear experts speak, see movies and slides on abdominal birth, and discuss your feelings with other parents who have had or are going to have cesarean babies—in all these ways you can help yourself to have the kind of birth experience you will be happy with.

Perhaps you will be able to ask for and get the kind of anesthesia you prefer. And maybe, if you are lucky, your husband will be allowed to accompany you into the delivery room and share your newborn's first moments of life with you. Perhaps you will be offered a chance to get acquainted with your infant right there on the delivery table, or even breast-feed in the recovery room. If you know what is in store and what your choices are, your newborn, if it is normal and healthy, may not have to be taken off to the intensive-care nursery and kept from you for at least a day and a night. It is possible you can have rooming-in after the first couple of days, and begin breast-feeding—if that is what you choose to do—the same day you deliver.

Even if you cannot manage to do everything the way you would choose, at least you will know what to look for next time around. You will know exactly what is going on and what is happening to you and your baby. Your natural fears of having a baby in this no-longer-so-unusual way will be diminished by the information you have gathered.

GREAT EXPECTATIONS FOR CHILDBIRTH

Paralleling the rise in the number of cesareans in the last ten years, there has been a sharp rise in expectations for the childbirth experience. The combination has been responsible for much of the emotional trauma that can result from an abdominal delivery, especially when it is unexpected.

Not very long ago, women expected little but travail from childbirth. They put themselves in the godlike hands of their obstetricians, wanting to know as little as possible about what was happening to them and to their bodies. "Wake me up when it's all over" was the typical attitude. But today many couples make plans to share the childbirth experience—with the mother fully conscious, undrugged, in control—participating as a team with the doctor in bringing forth their own new baby. They plan to go through a labor that is hard work (but eased by the relaxation techniques learned in prepared-childbirth classes), to be together for the delivery, to see and to hold their infant almost as soon as it is born, to form a family right there in the delivery room.

When these plans don't go as scheduled, when expectations aren't fulfilled, when the birthing is taken out of their hands and placed in those of a surgeon and an anonymous anesthesiologist, there is no way prepared parents are not going to be terribly disappointed. There is no way they won't feel cheated when they can't do what they had looked forward to, and perhaps glorified, during nine long months. Families are small today, and each birth becomes an event to be anticipated and savored.

Often cesarean parents, especially when they had built up a beautiful vision of what was going to happen, are more than disappointed—they are bereft. They have suffered a great loss, the loss of a "normal" delivery. Women frequently feel they have failed, done it "wrong," messed it up. Some consider themselves less of a woman; others are sure they have somehow brought this upon themselves, that it is their fault. At the very least, most women who had anticipated prepared childbirth seem to feel they have missed out on one of life's important experiences. They have a healthy baby, but all is not right.

Other people—husbands, parents, friends, hospital roommates—frequently add to these negative feelings because they, too, may look upon a cesarean birth as somehow unnatural and inferior. Or they imply you have done it "the easy way," you've "copped out."

Cesarean birth is neither inferior nor superior to a vaginal birth. Of course, one would prefer a simple vaginal birth because it is still the safest and easiest way to have a baby. But *cesarean birth is simply an alternative that is chosen when your well-being or your baby's well-being is threatened.* It is a medical necessity and a medical decision, one that you are in little position to dispute; nor could you avoid it through your own efforts at this moment. It is not "the easy way," nor does it represent a failure. But because the process of childbearing is so intertangled with self-image, a cesarean birth can easily turn out to be a psychological disaster even when it is an outstanding medical success.

Although most cesarean parents feel disappointed when they find out an abdominal birth is destined for them, and though the immediate recovery period is not as pleasant or rapid for the mother as it is with the usual birth, they accept the decision and its aftermath with some equanimity. Mothers manage to cope with the discomforts that accompany major surgery—especially if they know the basic facts and risks, have learned the best ways to deal with them, and receive sympathetic, loving care.

TURNING THE TIDE

Because more hospitals, obstetricians, and nurses, along with prepared-childbirth instructors, are now aware—chiefly because of consumer pressure—that cesarean parents want and deserve a happy birth experience just like other parents, they have begun to pay more attention to their needs. They are changing some of their traditional policies and routines, taking into consideration the emotional aspects of birth, and giving more intelligent and considerate postpartum care.

If the trend continues, as it certainly will, cesarean mothers will no longer be treated like "the section at the end of the hall," just another surgical patient, someone who is sick and weak, unable to function as other mothers do, separated from the birth experience, their husbands, and their babies.

Cesarean mothers, many of whom are in a hospital for the first time in their lives, usually have little idea of what to expect and what to ask for. As a result, their needs as new mothers are frequently ignored, even though the most important fact now is that a baby has been born.

Most women after a cesarean birth do not complain so much about the physical difficulties—which are acute for only two or three days—as about their fears, their confusion, their feelings of dehumanization, their loneliness, their anxieties about their babies, and their frustrated desires to begin acting like other new mothers without delay. They worry about being apart from their babies during their first days of life. They complain about their treatment in the hospital and the routinized care they may receive. In a recent survey made by Sheila La Frankie of the Westchester, New York, Chapter of ASPO,* the prepared-childbirth organization, only 10 percent of the cesarean mothers questioned reported they had had a satisfactory birth experience.

As the needs of cesarean parents, just like those of other parents, are beginning to be heeded, these experiences are changing.

* American Society of Psycho-Prophylaxis in Obstetrics.

The impact on obstetrics of the rising tide of consumerism has been significant, and prepared childbirth has played an increasingly large role in the way babies are being born. It has brought the parents into the decision-making, and has allowed them to assume responsibility for—and control over—much of what happens to them. Consumers have forced the medical profession to take hard looks at what it has always done quite routinely, and to make changes.

This hasn't always been easy, and sometimes the voices of change have become strident and certainly irritating to the establishment. Sometimes they aren't realistic, or practical. But they have brought about change that has long been needed.

At a time when the birthrate in the United States has significantly fallen and obstetrical services are vying for patients, the pressure of consumerism will clearly have an impact on which institutions and services will survive in the long run. It will noticeably affect which physicians are the busiest, and it has already stimulated the trend toward the use of nurse-midwives in normal, uncomplicated births.

The institutions and the physicians that are beginning to pay attention to their consumers will obviously become those chosen when there are alternatives. Unfortunately, in many parts of this country, there are no alternatives and little or no choice of doctor or hospital. But, even here, parents can have some influence on their own childbirth—when they make it known what they want.

Because cesarean parents *are* now making known what they want—good medical care *as well as* participation in the birth experience, early contact with their babies, and attention paid to their emotional needs as new parents—they are beginning to become part of the new way of having babies.

⊠ 2 ⊠

The Reason for Your Cesarean Birth

Primary (first-time) cesarean sections are seldom planned or even suspected in advance. In most cases, you go into the hospital after your labor begins, looking forward to having your baby just like everyone else you have ever known, and are surprised and disappointed, to put it mildly, when your doctor announces that you are going to have a cesarean birth.

Usually the decision is made after you have gone through at least a few hours of labor and sometimes many more, when it becomes apparent that the delivery is not progressing the way it should. The obstetrician decides that surgery is imperative in order to avoid the unnecessary trauma that might occur during a long and difficult labor and a complicated delivery—or perhaps even to save your life or your baby's.

The second time around, most cesarean births happen merely because the first one happened.

When you have an unplanned cesarean, the psychological impact may be devastating. You—and perhaps your husband—may have prepared yourselves to participate with the doctor in the usual kind of birth and you may be terribly unhappy when you can't do what you had planned to do. Not only that, but a true emergency cesarean almost always happens in an atmosphere of haste and tension, with little time for consideration of your feelings.

If this is the way it was with you, perhaps it will be helpful to discuss the reasons why some babies are delivered abdominally rather than in the usual way. None of these reasons is your "fault," any more than it's your fault that you have brown eyes or long legs. It isn't something you probably could have avoided by behaving or thinking differently; it doesn't mean you have done something wrong. The indication for your cesarean delivery is simply a physical fact, just as it is for an appendectomy.

Sometimes the indication for a surgical birth is "absolute," which means that normal labor and a vaginal delivery are impossible without endangering you or your baby, and there is no reasonable alternative. But sometimes the indications are "relative" and depend on the severity of your situation. A vaginal birth may be possible, but a cesarean section is deemed to be much safer. In this case, the decision is really a matter of judgment. Your obstetrician decides that it is too risky to wait or to take a chance on complications.

You, as the patient, will really take no part in this decision, which must be left to the medical experts. Nor is there usually time to call in a consultant. But remember that a baby born by cesarean will be just as healthy as a baby born in an uncomplicated vaginal delivery, and has *a far better chance* to be healthy than a baby who has a hard time making its way through the birth canal in a complicated delivery.

Sometimes the cesarean is performed because of a possible danger to you, and sometimes because the baby is in some sort of trouble. Often it's hard to separate the two, and frequently there is a combination of indications.

About 35 to 40 percent of first-time cesarean sections are done because of cephalopelvic disproportion or "failure to progress." About 10 percent are the result of hemorrhaging, while perhaps 20 percent take place because the baby is in an unusual position at term. Ten to 15 percent are performed because of "fetal distress," and the remainder happen because of various miscellaneous and rather rare circumstances.

PREVIOUS CESAREAN BIRTHS

About half of the cesarean births performed in the United States are "repeat sections," occurring simply because a mother has had a previous cesarean birth. Most obstetricians believe that once a woman has had an abdominal delivery she must not be allowed to labor or to give birth vaginally for fear of uterine rupture.

There is some difference of opinion about the need for *automatic* repeat cesarean deliveries and some cesarean mothers are now safely having babies in the traditional way—through the birth canal—after a normal labor. See Chapter 3 for a more detailed discussion of "once a cesarean, always a cesarean."

CEPHALOPELVIC DISPROPORTION

This is the most usual indication for a primary cesarean birth. It means that the baby's head (the biggest part of the baby) is too large to pass safely through your particular bony pelvic opening. Sometimes the baby is very large, maybe nine or ten pounds, and sometimes the pelvis is very small or unusually shaped, making even a six-pound baby too large to be comfortably born. This doesn't mean that every big baby must be delivered abdominally, or that every small pelvis requires an operation. Only a few women have pelvic structures so small that they can't deliver vaginally. But a combination of the two is definitely an absolute indication.

Usually there are additional factors that contribute to the decision to deliver by cesarean on the basis of cephalopelvic disproportion. These may include a failure of the labor to progress normally (when the uterine contractions are not sufficiently strong or effective to push the baby along quickly), as well as a malposition of the baby. A baby small enough to get through the birth canal when it presents the top of its head first may not be small enough if the presenting part is its buttocks or its face. A problem often occurs when the infant's head faces in the wrong direction (looking up rather than down); this may result in a long, arduous labor and delivery—or a cesarean section.

Though your doctor may suspect there is going to be disproportion, it is usually impossible to be sure until after labor has gone on for a while. When there is some question about the relative size of baby to pelvis, then your doctor may order tests. One is an X ray, which will show an outline of your pelvic structure, which can then be measured. This is called X-ray pelvimetry and is done during labor or, if a problem is suspected earlier, late in pregnancy. Using high-frequency sound waves (sonography), it is then possible to measure the diameter of the unborn baby's head (see Chapter 5). Together, the information gathered from the two tests allows a decision to be made about whether the baby is likely to be safely delivered "from below." Unfortunately, not every hospital has sonographic equipment available at all hours, and so these important data may not be there when they are needed.

FAILURE TO PROGRESS (DYSTOCIA) OR PROLONGED LABOR

Long labor can be totally exhausting for you and may become dangerous to your baby. Sometimes labor continues unabated for many hours but, because the uterine musculature fails to contract efficiently and completely, the cervix then fails to dilate as it should. Sometimes the baby's head refuses to descend into the pelvis. Sometimes the contractions are irregular both in interval and strength, and sometimes they stop altogether. Or they may not be strong enough. An active labor lasting longer than sixteen to eighteen hours is considered today to be risky to both you and your baby.

Failure to progress is not an absolute indication for cesarean birth, but it certainly is a reason to investigate what is going on. Once in a great while, severe anxiety will cause poor labor because of an outpouring of adrenal hormones. Most often, the cause will turn out to be cephalopelvic disproportion or malposition of the baby. But if it is determined that the baby is not too large for the pelvis, is in a deliverable position, and is at term, many physicians will decide to stimulate labor in the hope that this will move things along. And it usually does.

If there is still little or no progress after a few hours of stimulation, and especially if the amniotic membranes have ruptured, thus raising the possibility of infection, a cesarean may be the only way to proceed.

FETAL DISTRESS

Fetal distress is a major reason for unplanned cesarean sections. This term is another way of saying that the fetus may be suffering from hypoxia: that is, a reduced supply of oxygen. Fetal distress is signaled by changes in the fetal heart rate—usually a slowing of the rate *after* a contraction and continuing into the resting phase, sometimes a prolonged rapid beat, or unusual patterns of rate.

Not all changes in heart rate, and not all drops in rate, are ominous, and the beats are normally quite variable from beat to beat. Actually, checking the heart rate is rather like taking a temperature. The fact of a change does not mean that the baby is in jeopardy or even that it is sick. It is merely an indication that more investigation is needed. For example, minor degrees of cord compression, long contractions, and unequal pressure on the baby's head as it pushes against the cervix can all cause changes in the fetal heart rate, but none of them need have any real significance.

True fetal distress is almost always due to a markedly reduced flow of oxygen-rich blood to the baby. The most common causes are severe compression of the umbilical cord; diminished blood flow caused by cardiovascular disease of the mother; "premature aging of the placenta," which occurs in women whose diets have been very poor or who have diseases affecting the health of the blood vessels; severe infections; and, very rarely, chronic anxiety, which may constrict the blood vessels and so reduce the blood supply to the uterus.

One of the most accurate indications of reduced oxygen supply is a lowering of the pH of the baby's blood. The pH is a measure of the acidity or alkalinity of the blood. Too low a pH level, resulting from a reduced blood supply, is always a sign of trouble and means that the baby must be delivered quickly, perhaps by cesarean section. (A lowered fetal pH may also be a result of maternal disease, such as diabetic acidosis.) In many of our larger, more advanced medical centers, the baby's blood is always sampled whenever there is any sign of fetal distress.

If a pH is taken when the fetal heart monitor indicates

there may be problems, it is possible to diagnose fetal distress much more accurately. A cone-shaped speculum is inserted into the vagina, then moved up against the baby's head (or whatever other part of the baby may be presenting first) and a tiny nick is made in the scalp. A drop or two of blood is taken and quickly sampled for its concentration of oxygen and carbon dioxide, as well as its pH.

Fetal distress can also occur as a result of the elective induction of labor. When a delivery is scheduled in advance of the spontaneous onset of labor and the labor is induced artificially, sometimes the contractions are stimulated to occur almost continuously. Under these circumstances, the blood supply to the baby is almost always reduced. Then, because the mother is so uncomfortable with her unrelenting contractions with no time in between to rest, she may be given an epidural anesthesia to numb the feeling in her lower body. This may further reduce her blood pressure, resulting in fetal distress and a cesarean section.

When true fetal distress becomes apparent toward the end of labor, the obstetrician will try to deliver the baby by the vaginal route as quickly and safely as possible. But when it happens early and the labor looks as though it will continue for many more hours, the only way to deliver the baby fast enough is by cesarean.

The use of electronic fetal heart monitors has often been blamed for the increase in the incidence of cesarean deliveries for fetal distress. Before monitors, physicians or nurses listened to the baby's heartbeat every fifteen minutes or so. But with the machines, which chart the contractions as well as the heartbeat, doctors can get a much closer insight into what is going on inside the uterus.

An external monitor consists of a belt worn around your abdomen while you are in labor. It isn't uncomfortable and can be easily removed. Sometimes, when a closer investigation of the fetus is desired, and when the membranes have already ruptured, an internal monitor is also used because it provides a much more accurate reading of the heart rate. A small clip is inserted through the vagina and superficially attached to the baby's scalp. The infant may have a small mark on its head for a few days after birth, but this mark is never permanent and the procedure is quite safe.

Monitoring has become the subject of much controversy in obstetrics. Many people denounce the proliferation of electronic equipment in the labor room as dehumanizing, and they claim that it causes unnecessary intervention—such as cesarean sections—in what might otherwise be normal, safe births. It is true that the monitors have helped to increase the number of cesareans performed in this country, some of them totally unnecessary. On the other hand, there is no question that continuous monitoring provides much more reliable information about the state of the fetus than we could ever get with our hands and our ears, and that the monitors have saved many babies from permanent damage resulting from a long, hard labor without an adequate oxygen supply.

When monitors are correctly interpreted, they can be invaluable tools. They can spot abnormalities in the earliest stages, and they can take much of the guesswork out of obstetrics. The problem is that physicians and nurses sometimes do not fully understand the information they are getting from the machines. Sometimes they are not yet expert at distinguishing between a perfectly normal, though unusual, heart rate and one that spells trouble. Whenever an abnormality is suspected, doctors tend to feel that it is safer to perform surgery than to take a chance that all will go well. As we said before, a major reason why this happens with increasing frequency is the fear of malpractice suits. With a permanent printout of contractions and heart rate, many doctors are afraid *not* to do a cesarean, even when the record does not clearly indicate true fetal distress.

Another problem, as we have said, is that the monitors are not infallible. They can misfunction, sending out quite misleading information which, because of the possible urgency of the situation, can lead to surgery that might have been avoided.

Unfortunately, there is nothing you, as an obstetrical patient in the hospital ready to have your baby, can do to prevent a perhaps unnecessary cesarean section. You can't shout, "Stop! I insist that we wait an hour to make sure this operation is really needed!" When you are told you must have surgery if you want a live, healthy baby, you cannot take the chance that it may not be true. But the fact is that never before have so many babies been delivered by cesarean section because of "fetal distress," many of them turning out to be normal infants who show no signs of such distress. Fetal distress is diagnosed far more often than it actually exists.

Despite the drawbacks, however, fetal heart monitors *should always be available* in every hospital in case they are needed because they do provide more accurate information than we can get without them. As the monitors become more common and medical personnel become more expert in interpreting their results, fewer cesarean sections will be performed unnecessarily.

ABNORMAL POSITIONS

Ideally, your baby will make its entrance into the world in the vertex position. This means that it will come down the birth canal head first, with its chin bent down on its chest and its face toward your backbone. This is the way it will pass most easily through the pelvis—with its head gradually molding itself during your labor to the size and shape of the opening.

Sometimes, however, the baby won't be so accommodating and will decide to arrive buttocks or feet first. This is called a breech presentation, or a breech birth. Many first breech babies can be delivered normally, with perhaps a little more difficulty and concern than is usual. But often a doctor will judge that a cesarean section is the safest way for a breech baby to be born. Today 30 to 40 percent of all breech babies in this country are delivered abdominally because cesarean deliveries have become so much less risky.

Less frequently, the baby will arrive face first, or brow first, or perhaps its shoulder will be the presenting part, or even both a hand and a foot. These abnormal positions may also require a cesarean delivery.

Each case must be judged individually when there is a breech position. If you have a roomy pelvis and are having a good strong labor, and if the baby is in a frank breech presentation (the baby is flexed at the hips, with its feet up at its head, and comes down rear end first) and is of average size, then there is usually no reason for surgery. The chief concern is whether the baby's head is small enough to pass safely through the pelvis.

Much depends on the skill, experience, and judgment of your obstetrician, as well as the use of the sophisticated tools available today. If there is any question about the relative size of the baby's head to your pelvis—and there is always some question when this is your first baby and your pelvis has never been "tested"—then there are X-ray machines to measure the dimensions of the pelvis and sonograms to give the dimensions and position of the baby.

With a breech delivery, the head comes out last and, obviously, we must be sure it will readily deliver. When there is any doubt, a cesarean birth is the wisest choice. The best time for the cesarean is just after labor has begun on its own and the baby has attained its full maturity.

An interesting note: many babies are not in the head-first vertex position even a few weeks before term, but about 96 percent of all full-term infants turn around by the time labor begins.

PREMATURE BREECH BABIES

Even if your pelvis is adequately large, many obstetricians today will perform a cesarean for the delivery of a premature breech baby. Of course, this happens only when premature labor has been established and cannot be stopped, making delivery inevitable. Recent data have shown that a cesarean delivery is best for babies at twenty-eight to thirty-two weeks if they are in a breech position, because they are so very fragile at this stage of development. Many obstetricians feel, however, that a vaginal delivery is fine if the baby is descending headfirst.

TRANSVERSE LIE

Occasionally, when labor begins, a baby will be in a transverse position. This means that it is lying *across* the abdomen with its head on one side and its feet on the other. There is no way a baby in this position can possibly be delivered through the vagina, and a cesarean is always the only solution.

HEMORRHAGE

Hemorrhaging from the uterus is one of the major causes of emergency cesareans, and the most dramatic. If it occurs, it means your baby will be delivered in tremendous haste to avoid excessive blood loss both to you and to the baby. This can truly be a matter of life and death.

There are two common causes of uterine hemorrhage. One is placenta previa, which means that the placenta, which is normally found at the top of the uterus, is abnormally implanted in the lower segment, blocking the baby's exit and giving it no way to get out. As labor progresses and the cervix begins to thin out (efface) and dilate, the attachment of the placenta breaks away from the walls of the uterus, tearing the multitude of blood vessels from the placenta to the maternal blood supply. Studies have shown that having a previous cesarean delivery increases your chances of having a placenta previa in your subsequent pregnancies.

Fortunately, a placenta previa is often detected early, long before any difficulties begin. Most women with this condition have a few episodes of vaginal bleeding, starting at about thirty-two weeks of pregnancy. If placenta previa is suspected, probably the best way to make a diagnosis is by sonography (see page 51), which will make a "picture" showing the presence and location of the misplaced placenta.

If the placenta is centrally located, lying directly over the opening of the cervix, then a cesarean delivery is absolutely essential. If it only partially blocks the birth canal, a vaginal delivery may still be possible. This depends on the amount of bleeding and how much of the placenta is lying over the cervical opening.

The other common cause of hemorrhaging is abruptio placentae, the premature separation of a normally implanted placenta from the uterine wall. This kind of uterine hemorrhage is often associated with toxemia of pregnancy, hypertensive diseases, and "advanced maternal age." In some ways, abruptio placentae can be a more threatening situation than a placenta previa because, when the normal attachments come apart, blood sometimes fills up the space between, cutting off the blood supply to the fetus.

Even so, there is a wide margin of safety. Almost half of the placenta can detach and there will still be enough transfer of blood and oxygen across the surfaces to assure the birth of a healthy baby.

Depending on just how much of an abruption has occurred, a cesarean may or may not be needed. If the bleeding becomes heavy and the baby is not going to deliver quickly, a cesarean is the usual course of action.

CORD ACCIDENTS

Sudden and severe fetal distress can be caused by an accident involving the umbilical cord. The cord is normally about two feet long, connects the baby to the placenta, and carries all of the baby's blood supply from the mother. In some rare cases, however, it gets in the way of the delivery. It may prolapse, which means it pops through the birth canal first and is then squeezed by the baby's head or shoulder as the infant descends into the pelvis. A compressed cord means the baby suddenly gets less blood and oxygen than it needs.

A very short umbilical cord may constrict circulation as the baby moves down into the pelvis, stretching the cord as it goes. And a particularly long cord may wrap around the baby or knot or tangle, again cutting off circulation. (Quite commonly, though, the cord will wrap around the baby's neck and cause no difficulty at all or only a transient slowing of the heart.)

When any of these complications happens—and they are *very rare*—an emergency cesarean is usually performed in a hurry.

MULTIPLE GESTATION

The use of various fertility drugs has quite significantly increased the number of unusual multiple births. Such pregnancies present many difficult problems for the mother and the obstetrician, including the manner of delivery. Most physicians consider it safest to deliver three or more babies by cesarean section. The infants are almost always premature, and the positions the babies assume in the uterus can be astounding.

FIBROIDS OR TUMORS

Extremely rarely, a uterine fibroid will obstruct the birth canal so the fetus cannot make its way through. The fibroid is usually discovered early in the pregnancy and a cesarean section is planned long in advance.

"ADVANCED MATERNAL AGE"

Not many years ago, one of the common reasons a woman had a cesarean birth was simply that she was over thirty-five years of age. It was thought that a woman of such "advanced" years was not in shape to go through the trauma of labor and delivery. But trends in obstetrics are changing. Many women are now electing to have their first child relatively late in life, perhaps after establishing a career. Doctors now realize that these women, when they are in good health, are no more in need of a cesarean delivery than any other normal pregnant woman. A healthy forty-year-old woman, for example, even having her first baby, does not require an abdominal delivery simply because she is forty.

However, her age is one more factor to consider when there are other problems. If there is a marginal risk of some sort—perhaps a breech baby or the possibility of a moderate amount of disproportion between mother and baby—most doctors would perform a cesarean in order to avoid taking even that slight chance that something might go wrong. Their decision would usually be based on the fact that this woman does not have many years of child-bearing capacity ahead of her.

Also, by the time any one of us reaches the age of forty or forty-two, we may have acquired medical problems. Certain of them could complicate the course of a pregnancy and make a cesarean section a necessity.

MATERNAL DISEASE

There are a very few maternal diseases that may make a cesarean delivery likely, though even when these diseases are present, most deliveries can still be done vaginally with very careful supervision. However, when the disease has affected the uterine blood supply, the ability of the uterus to contract, or the ability to sustain the work load of hours of active labor, then a cesarean must be performed. Sometimes the disease may pose a threat to the infant because the poor condition of the mother's cardiovascular system results in a reduced supply of oxygen and nutrients to the baby, and perhaps a diminished removal rate of metabolic waste products. The infant may not grow as well as it should within the uterus. This is called "intrauterine growth retardation." And sometimes the baby cannot stand the stresses of either a normal or an induced labor.

Diabetes

The diabetic woman who is dependent upon supplementary insulin runs the risk of losing her baby if she is allowed to go to term and start labor spontaneously, particularly if her blood sugar has not been rigidly controlled. The incidence of stillborns with diabetic mothers who reach term is over 20 percent. Therefore, the birth is almost always planned to take place at some time before the full nine months are up. This doesn't necessarily mean that if you are an insulin-dependent diabetic you will have to have a cesarean, but it is a very good possibility.

The way the baby is delivered depends on several factors. If all the special tests now available for determining the maturity of the fetus (see Chapter 5) have indicated that the time is at hand for delivery, if the fetus seems healthy, the head is in the pelvis, and the cervix is ready, then the baby may be born vaginally after labor has been induced.

If, however, none of these factors is in your favor, and if it looks as if the alternative to cesarean section might be a very lengthy induction, which may take one or two or maybe three days and can be dangerous both to the baby and to the diabetic mother, then a quick abdominal birth is much better.

There is a separate group of women who are called "class A diabetics" or "gestational diabetics" because their diabetes is evident only during pregnancy. These women simply require careful observation during pregnancy, labor, and delivery. They do not have to be induced early, unless there is some reason to think that the baby is in danger.

Also, any woman who has had children *before* becoming diabetic and pregnant again stands a good chance of having her labor induced successfully and of avoiding a cesarean birth.

Recent work at the Sosnoff Diabetic Service at Mt. Sinai Medical Center in New York and other medical institutions indicates that women who can maintain *rigid* control of their blood sugar during their pregnancies greatly increase their chances of carrying their babies to full term and going into spontaneous labor. They can also greatly reduce their risk of having a very large baby. So, in both these ways, with strict control they can often manage to deliver vaginally, avoiding the need for surgery.

Rigid control means just that. Blood-sugar levels must be maintained within the normal limits of a normal non-diabetic pregnant woman. This is certainly not easy, but it can be done with the constant attention of the obstetrician, the diabetologist, and you.

If your diabetes can be controlled by diet alone, you may get along very well by simply watching what you eat and staying in close touch with your doctors. Or you may need insulin temporarily because you won't produce enough yourself to satisfy the huge demands of a pregnancy.

If you are normally controlled by diet plus oral hypoglycemic agents, you must now switch to insulin until after the baby is born because the oral agents will not only stimulate your pancreas to produce insulin but the baby's as well.

An insulin-dependent diabetic must closely monitor her blood sugar several times a day, testing the level in the *blood* rather than the urine. The blood-sugar level can be tested with chemically treated plastic strips called Chemstrips, or by Dextrostix and a relatively inexpensive machine—a reflectance meter—that provides a more accurate reading than your eye can possibly manage.

In response to the blood-sugar levels, insulin must be injected *at least* twice a day, more likely three or four times a day, in split doses, with regular insulin added just before each meal. Many women find that using an insulin pump throughout their pregnancies is an even easier way to make sure they receive the proper amounts of insulin all day long.

And you must see your doctor about three times a week.

Is it worth all the hard work to maintain such rigid control? It definitely is, because it means you can have your baby much more safely and perhaps without needing a cesarean delivery. Besides, with excellent blood-sugar control, you may well discover that your general health is greatly improved as well. Such results may encourage you to keep up the good work.

Hypertension

Chronic high blood pressure is another disease that may require a cesarean delivery because it affects the cardiovascular system and tends to narrow and constrict the blood vessels. When the arteries cannot deliver the normal flow of blood to the uterus, then there is always the danger that the baby will be threatened by the stresses of labor.

Toxemia of Pregnancy (Pre-eclampsia)

For reasons that are not totally understood, some women late in pregnancy develop toxemia. This is a condition characterized by sudden heightened blood pressure, significant amounts of protein in the urine, and excessive fluid retention, which causes marked swelling, particularly of the face and the extremities. Sometimes toxemia can be controlled by medication, but sometimes it can become a serious threat to both mother and the baby because of a diminished fetal blood supply.

When this happens, the answer is to deliver the baby as quickly as possible. If labor can be safely induced, a vaginal delivery is perfectly fine; if it cannot, a cesarean delivery is the wisest course to take.

Heart Disease

Cesarean births for women with serious heart disease have become quite uncommon today, and there are few situations where surgery is the preferred method of delivery. The threat, in this case, is not to the baby but to the mother, and good anesthetic techniques have been developed in recent years that will protect her from the stresses of labor.

RH Disease (*Erythroblastosis Fetalis*)

When a woman whose blood is typed Rh-negative gives birth to a Rh-positive baby, she may become sensitized to the blood of her future Rh-positive babies, causing serious problems for these infants. However, thanks to a vaccine called Rhogam, Rh incompatibility is a disease that is rapidly disappearing in this country. This vaccine, when given to the mother within seventy-two hours of the delivery of her first baby, will keep her from becoming sensitized in the future. But the incompatibility still occurs occasionally. Sometimes, when the fetus is endangered by anemia as a result and the delivery cannot be induced safely and successfully, a cesarean will be needed.

FAILED ELECTIVE INDUCTION

Some cesareans are performed because of "failed" elective inductions—and the result is often a premature baby. When there is an induction, which means that labor is initiated by drugs on a prearranged date, it is obvious that the calculations of the proper time for delivery can be wrong. If you are induced and do not dilate as expected after about five hours, it means you are probably not ready for labor and it is too early for the baby to be born.

If the amniotic membranes have not been ruptured, the induction may be interrupted and you may be allowed to wait for labor to begin spontaneously at a later time. But if they have ruptured, it is too late to turn back. So a cesarean becomes necessary to finish the job of delivery.

If your doctor decides upon an elective induction for a valid reason (which should *not* be his golf schedule or your possible tax savings), the essential maturity tests should be made first (see Chapter 5).

PROLONGED RUPTURED MEMBRANES

When their babies are at term and the cervix is ready to dilate, the vast majority of women—well over 90 percent—go into labor spontaneously within twenty-four to forty-eight hours after their membranes rupture. But after about twenty-four hours of waiting for labor to begin by itself, most obstetricians will decide it is wise to induce labor because of the distinct possibility that an intrauterine infection might develop.

If a vaginal delivery does not seem likely after three or four hours of induced labor, the doctor will probably elect to perform a cesarean to protect the baby from the dangers of infection. This indication for cesarean delivery is called "prolonged ruptured membranes and a failed induction."

If the membranes rupture prematurely, then the decisions involved are much more complex. If there is a reasonable chance that the fetus is mature enough to survive outside the mother's body, most obstetricians will go ahead and induce labor and/or perform a cesarean. If, on the other hand, it is still too early for the baby to be born safely and there is no evidence of infection, many doctors would prefer to monitor the situation carefully and allow the pregnancy to continue as long as possible. Without infection, it is better to leave the baby in the uterus to thrive and grow. With infection, however, delivery is imperative.

UNUSUAL INDICATIONS FOR
CESAREAN DELIVERY

If you have had extensive surgery on your uterus (such as a hysterotomy, or the removal of very large fibroids that required an incision into the uterine cavity, or a metroplasty to rebuild a deformed uterus), which has left a large and perhaps fragile scar, cesarean section is almost always the best method of delivery for you.

Occasionally, previous vaginal surgery, as well as surgical repair of the bladder or rectum, is also a valid indication for a cesarean. A cesarean delivery avoids the stretching and trauma to these organs that a vaginal birth would involve.

HERPES INFECTION

An acute case of herpes genitalis—a sexually transmitted viral disease that has become almost epidemic in the last five years—is an absolute indication for cesarean section. When there are open herpes lesions in the cervix or vagina, it would be most dangerous to allow the baby to pass through the birth canal. The herpes virus is extremely toxic; it can cause an overwhelming generalized infection, a high fever, or perhaps brain damage or even death in a newborn baby. If the infection is not in the acute stage, however, and there are no open lesions, your doctor may feel it is safe to deliver the baby in the traditional way.

The indications for allowing a vaginal delivery when you have herpes are generally defined this way: 1. there has been no evidence of primary disease for four weeks; 2. there have been no recurrent lesions for two weeks; 3. no lesions are visible at the time labor begins; and 4. the results of a vaginal culture are negative.

Most physicians today have facilities in their offices for culturing the herpes virus. If you aren't certain whether you have ever had herpes, then a serological test may provide the information. This is important, because about 10 percent of all babies born with neonatal herpes are born to women who are unaware they have the disease. If you have a history of a herpetic genital infection, you should have a herpes culture in the last few weeks of pregnancy and, of course, should report any recurrences immediately to your doctor.

POST-MATURITY

When a normal pregnancy continues for more than two weeks beyond the calculated due date, the usual explanation is that the calculations were wrong. Occasionally, though, the date is quite correct and the prolonged pregnancy may represent a distinct threat to the unborn infant's life. This situation requires careful monitoring. If there is any suggestion of real danger to the health of the baby waiting in the uterus, your doctor will probably try to induce labor. If this doesn't work out as planned, you will have a cesarean birth.

☒ 3 ☒

Once a Cesarean,
Always a Cesarean?

There is no real physical limit to the number of cesarean births you can have. Ethel Kennedy, for instance, has had eleven of them. It has been traditional in this country, though, to have three cesarean births and then, during the last one, to be sterilized. Many doctors feel that three major abdominal operations are plenty for any woman. This is not necessarily so. If you are willing to have another major operation, there is no reason why you cannot have as many children as you wish (eleven may be going a little far). You should, however, be aware that each delivery may become somewhat more difficult because of the buildup of scar tissue and perhaps adhesions.

For most women, there is no reason to wait any longer between pregnancies after a cesarean birth than after a non-surgical birth, since your scar is normally completely healed within a couple of months. Most obstetricians advise waiting about a year before becoming pregnant again, but this is probably because they believe in giving you plenty of time to recover from a major operation before having another. If you feel well and did not have complications after the first birth, and if your doctor agrees that it is quite safe in your case, there is no real requirement to wait that long if you don't want to.

Your future fertility is rarely affected by having a cesarean birth.

GOING INTO LABOR BEFORE A REPEAT CESAREAN

If you are having a repeat cesarean delivery (which means you are preparing for your second or more surgical birth) and the plan is to deliver the baby *before* labor begins, what should you do if you think you are having contractions? Call your doctor immediately. It is never too soon—no matter how the contractions are spaced or whether you think they may be false labor—to notify the obstetrician. He or she may send you promptly to the hospital.

You should report not only labor, but also ruptured membranes or "bloody show" without delay. If you have already had a cesarean birth, *do not* labor at home. Go immediately to the hospital, where you will be under careful supervision.

Many physicians do not schedule cesarean births, but purposely allow their patients to go into labor first. This is so that they will be as sure as possible that the baby is mature. If that is your plan, call your doctor to let him/her know just as soon as the contractions begin.

By the way, contractions do not interfere with the surgery.

POSSIBLE DANGER SIGNS BEFORE A PLANNED OR REPEAT CESAREAN BIRTH

If at any time during your pregnancy you have *any* unexplained and persistent abdominal pain, or *any* vaginal bleeding, report to your obstetrician without delay. It may have no real significance at all, or it may mean your cesarean birth will happen before you thought it would. Don't try to make the decision yourself about whether your symptoms are important, and don't worry about needlessly bothering the doctor. Call.

Is a Vaginal Delivery Possible Now?

If you have had one baby by cesarean section, does that mean all your subsequent children must be delivered the same way? Or is it possible and safe to deliver vaginally the next time around?

The conservative and traditional medical point of view has always followed Dr. E. B. Cragin's edict stated back in 1916: "Once a cesarean, always a cesarean." This view holds that after a cesarean has been performed, once a uterus has been incised and is now scarred, it is too dangerous, because of the risk of rupture, to allow that uterus to labor sufficiently to deliver in the usual way.

Today it is still not a simple matter to find a physician who is willing to consider the possibility of a vaginal delivery after a cesarean.

This does not mean that it cannot be done and, in fact, *there is no valid reason* why you must have a repeat cesarean simply because you have had one before. What matters is the reason for the previous abdominal delivery, as well as the kind of incision that was made. A large and growing number of physicians today do not feel that, because you have had a first cesarean, you necessarily have to have another. In the last few years, more and more women who have had cesareans are searching for, and finding, doctors who will deliver their babies in the usual way when it is feasible in their case.

Many women want desperately to go through labor and delivery and to avoid the sometimes unpleasant and uncomfortable subsequences of major surgery that put them out of commission temporarily and may take some of the joy out of childbirth. To some women—especially those who have dutifully trained themselves for natural childbirth before their first deliveries and were terribly disappointed when they were not able to push out their own babies—a vaginal birth is of extreme importance. They want to go through what they consider to be a "normal" birth. To others, the issue is not vital. They are willing and able to accept the fact that, for them, childbirth will always mean surgery.

Probably, most women do not even know that a vaginal delivery is possible after a cesarean. Some are not willing to take the slight risk that it may incur, and some, in the face of the prevalent medical attitudes, are not strongly enough motivated to insist that their doctor consider them for a vaginal delivery. Others prefer the prospect of not having to go through labor, especially if their last one was difficult. And many women want to *know* what is going to happen—they do not want eight or nine months of uncertainty about whether or not they will be able to go through with a vaginal birth, and then perhaps not find out until after labor has begun.

And, of course, there are some women for whom it would be totally impossible to deliver vaginally the second or third time around, just as it was the first time.

When a vaginal delivery is possible and safe, it is better than a cesarean—whether or not you have had a surgical delivery before. Not only is it usually much more emotionally satisfying, but it may be *safer* than a cesarean. Even though a cesarean section is one of the safest surgical operations performed today, it is still a major operation. It isn't less major the second or the third time than the first, and the risks are generally the same. Not many women get wound infections after a cesarean, for example, but none would get a wound infection without a wound.

Anesthesia has become extremely safe, but it is always best to avoid it if you can.

So there are medical reasons why it is preferable to have a vaginal birth, if it is not contraindicated in your case.

IF YOU WANT A VAGINAL DELIVERY

First, we must assume that you can find an obstetrician who is willing to consider you for such a delivery. This may take time, perhaps money for consultation fees, and powerful motivation. You may have to shop around, and interview many doctors—weighing their words and their reputations as you go—before you find one who is willing, who understands your feelings, and whom you trust.

Not every obstetrician can even comprehend why a vaginal delivery may be important to you. The attitude often is "All you should be interested in is having a healthy baby. Why take a chance? What difference does it make?" Cesarean section has become so safe today that many doctors can't understand the desire of many women to be, in their own words, "normal," "whole," "successful," "intact." They can't understand it any more than they can understand the desire of a forty-two-year-old woman to keep her uterus when she has fibroids that must be removed. To her, it is an essential part of her femininity. They think, "What for? You won't need it anymore."

If you don't want to have an *automatic* subsequent cesarean, you must find a doctor who can understand your emotional need to have your baby just like most other women, no matter how irrational the need may sound to someone who hasn't experienced abdominal childbirth.

Some physicians today even suggest to certain of their patients that a vaginal delivery is possible for them—if they want it. Most women *don't* want it. They prefer to be able to plan the birth, to arrange for their other children at home, to avoid having to make such a momentous decision. The women who *do* wish to give vaginal birth a try are invariably those who took their prepared-childbirth classes very seriously and were shattered when their plans went awry the first or second time around.

The physician who refuses to consider a vaginal delivery for you may have many reasons for this decision. First, perhaps there is a medically valid reason why it would not be safe for you (see below). He (she) may honestly believe that "once a cesarean, always a cesarean" is the safest policy. Or he may be more concerned with possible malpractice suits than with what you want. He may not feel comfortable delivering a baby from a previously incised uterus. He may never have done it before or seen it done and will approach the idea with trepidation.

THE PREREQUISITES FOR A SAFE DELIVERY

The doctor must deliver the baby in a *fully equipped* medical center where, if a cesarean section becomes the necessary route after attempting to deliver vaginally—and this is always a possibility—there will be no delay in performing the operation.

Even in New York City, there are hospitals where, if a decision is made to perform a cesarean, the baby may not be delivered for an hour. That may be too long. These are not the hospitals in which a cesarean mother should attempt a vaginal delivery. You must know in advance that if anything should go wrong during the labor (rare but possible), you can have a cesarean immediately. The safety factor must be present. That means a full-time staff, a full-time operating room, and a full-time anesthesiologist ready to go in a hurry. It means a good twenty-four-hour blood bank with cross-matched blood ready for you just in case it's needed. And it means, where possible, an operating room on the same floor as the labor room.

Because a trial of labor for a woman who has had a

previous cesarean requires the full array of medical facilities and personnel, it would be an excellent idea—if you were planning to have your baby at a small community hospital without these facilities—for your obstetrician to arrange a transfer to a larger institution where they are available

If you do not have the same obstetrician who delivered you the first time, your doctor must be able to see your old hospital records. He (she) should never wholly depend on the information you provide—patients tend to have faulty memories for specific medical data, and perhaps you were never told exactly why or how your delivery was made. The details surrounding your previous cesarean birth—the causes, the course of the delivery, and the postoperative recovery—are all vital if a wise decision is to be made now.

The next prerequisite for a vaginal delivery after an earlier cesarean is the *constant presence* of the physician. The doctor must be there with you from the moment you enter the hospital in labor until after the baby is safely delivered and the uterus is manually explored to be sure the scar is intact. He (she) must not turn you over to a resident or obstetrical nurse with instructions to call him when you are eight centimeters dilated and ready to go. This is another reason why physicians frequently object to attempting a vaginal delivery. Instead of spending the time in the office seeing other patients while you are laboring, the physician must spend many hours exclusively with you, at a time that may be totally inconvenient. Your delivery may take as long as ten hours out of the doctor's day—or night—while a repeat cesarean would take only an hour or so.

WHY DID YOU HAVE YOUR CESAREAN?

The very first consideration in weighing the chances of a successful vaginal delivery is the reason for the previous cesarean. Was it a "repeating" reason or a "nonrepeating" one? If it was repeating, which means the original cause is still present, the likelihood of a successful vaginal delivery is somewhat diminished but not impossible. As more and more women are given a trial of labor after a previous cesarean, a significant number of those whose surgery was performed because of cephalopelvic disproportion (see page 13) are successfully delivering vaginally. Furthermore, they sometimes deliver even *larger* babies than the ones they had by cesarean the first time.

Of course, if you go into premature labor, at, say, seven and a half months, when the fetus is only three and a half to four pounds, vaginal delivery may be quite easy and safe. Once again, some physicians would prefer to deliver a premature breech baby by cesarean.

Chances are, too, that if the reason for the first cesarean was chronic hypertension, heart disease, or diabetes, you will need a surgical delivery again.

If, however, your first cesarean occurred because of fetal distress, placenta previa, abruptio placentae, toxemia, infection, malposition, or multiple gestation, the chances are very good that this condition will not occur the next time and you may be a candidate for a vaginal delivery. Each of these causes is not permanent and not likely to be present another time. It was simply an accident.

The second important consideration, when you are eager to have a vaginal delivery for your second or third baby, is the kind of uterine incision you had before. Did you have a classical (vertical) incision through the upper part of the uterus, or did you have a low-flap transverse (horizontal) incision? By the way, the visible scar on your abdomen does not necessarily match the incision on your uterus. Since you could have had a "bikini" skin incision and a classical uterine incision, your doctor must consult the medical records to be certain.

Years ago, when most cesarean sections were done with

a classical incision, uterine rupture in subsequent labors was always a distinct possibility (about 2 percent) and a serious matter. A classical incision is still not considered a good risk for future vaginal delivery.

But the incidence of uterine rupture prior to or during labor from a low-flap transverse scar is small. The risk of a ruptured uterus with this incision is about 0.5 percent, and the risk of an incomplete rupture, or separation of the uterine wall rather like a hernia, is only slightly greater and is seldom cause for concern.

The uterus has an almost infinite capacity to stretch and can contain as much as fifteen to eighteen pounds of baby, placenta, cord, and amniotic fluid. The idea that the uterus has less capacity to stretch because it has a scar in it is not really valid. Many doctors have never seen a lower uterine scar rupture, but some still fear it enough to prefer to deliver all subsequent babies surgically.

Though the risk is small, attention must be paid to the scar during pregnancy to be sure it isn't in danger of separating, and certainly during labor, when disruption or separation may be indicated by tenderness or persistent and unusual pain between contractions in the area of the old uterine scar.

YOUR PART IN THE DECISION

Let's assume that you have found an obstetrician who is willing to deliver you vaginally if this is possible, who will do it in a well-equipped hospital with twenty-four-hour coverage, who understands why this is so important to you, and who wholeheartedly believes this kind of birth is best if it can be accomplished. What is your role?

First, you must be prepared to take some responsibility when you make the decision to try it. It is very important that you do not have significant amounts of anesthesia or analgesia while you are in labor. So you must learn the techniques of prepared childbirth, attend classes regularly, and be ready to have "natural" childbirth with little or no medication.

The reason for this is that you must be able to clearly feel any unusual pain or discomfort between contractions. A small dose of pain medication, if it is needed, will not mask any unusual pain, but heavy medication or anesthesia will, and so must not be given. If you cannot manage to go through the labor and delivery without much medication, then your doctor will probably decide to perform another cesarean.

If the doctor detects tenderness or persistent pain in the uterus between contractions or if there is bleeding—which may be the outward signs of an impending ruptured scar— then a cesarean will definitely be mandatory. The risk is tiny with a low-flap transverse scar, but it is always a possibility. So if you opt for a vaginal delivery, you must be willing to take that gamble. If it happens in a hospital where all the necessary safeguards are available—in other words, where the cesarean, if it becomes necessary, can be performed quickly and safely—the likelihood of trouble is quite small.

Though there are some risks in trying for a vaginal delivery, they should not be sufficient to dissuade most normal, healthy women from going through with it. Opinions obviously differ, however, and the decision must be discussed in great detail among woman, husband, and doctor.

YOU MAY TRY AND NOT SUCCEED

The other risk you face when trying for a vaginal delivery following an earlier cesarean is that you may again be disappointed. You may once more need an abdominal birth if, again, circumstances dictate it. And the decision may not be made until almost the last minute. No physician, for example, no matter how anxious he (or she) is to give a patient what she wants, would attempt to deliver a nine-pound baby in a breech position to a woman whose uterus was previously incised. Nor would he if the labor fails to progress in a normal fashion because of a large baby or a malposition.

How It Will Probably Happen

Before making the final decision to try for a vaginal delivery, your physician may order X-ray pelvimetry (X rays of the pelvic bones) unless you have once vaginally delivered a large baby. This will help to estimate your pelvic capacity. And, if sonography is available in your hospital, the doctor will also get pictures of the baby's head after you have begun labor in order to make the best decision. Your labor and contractions will undoubtedly be monitored electronically.

You will probably be allowed to go into spontaneous labor, and then intently watched to see how you progress. Most doctors will somewhat arbitrarily choose a number of hours of labor, with the expectation that a normal delivery will then occur.

Though most obstetricians hesitate to give oxytocin (the drug that stimulates uterine contractions) to women who have had earlier cesareans, many others, including myself, feel that, when there is no contraindication to normal labor, then there is no contraindication to the use of oxytocin either. As in any other vaginal delivery, the drug must be closely controlled in both duration and intensity of effect.

If you are laboring well, with progressive dilatation of the cervix along with progressive descent of the baby into the birth canal, and you will obviously deliver soon, fine. If, however, it appears that delivery is still many hours away, after, say, eight hours of labor, then the decision will probably be made that a cesarean is the route to take. All physicians must reserve the right to change their minds in midstream, to do what is most comfortable for them and safest for you and your baby.

✳ 4 ✳

Does a Cesarean Delivery
Affect Your Baby?

A baby delivered by cesarean section goes through a birth process that is mechanically very different from the usual birth. Its transition into the world is much more abrupt, and it skips the prolonged squeezing and pressure other babies go through during labor and passage through the birth canal. Usually, for anywhere between two and fifteen hours, most newborns' heads are used as battering rams, molding and reshaping until they reach the outside world. This doesn't happen with a cesarean baby, except, to some degree, if there has been a long labor before surgery.

No one yet knows whether arriving by cesarean has any significant or lasting effect on a newborn baby, but there is no hard evidence to demonstrate that there is any difference at all between a normal cesarean baby and a normal baby born in a nontraumatic vaginal delivery. Of course, cesarean babies are always in better condition than they would have been had they gone through a very difficult forceps or breech delivery.

In general, with today's major improvements in obstetrics and newborn care, infants delivered surgically do well and seem to suffer no disabilities as the result of their particular route into the world.

There has been much speculation that these babies are psychologically different from other infants, that they are affected in some subtle way by the more abrupt transition. There are no scientific facts to document this. Undoubtedly there is a psychological effect on a baby delivered by cesarean section whose parents' attitude toward it is affected by the very fact of the method of delivery. Frequently—however untrue—parents assume their baby is fragile, perhaps even sickly, just because it arrived this way, and so the baby is treated differently from a baby born in the usual fashion.

Sometimes a mother will react with some hostility and apprehension toward an infant whose birth necessitated a major assault on her body and its subsequent discomforts. This can cause a lasting effect on her feelings toward her baby. Also, the separation of mother and baby that often occurs after a cesarean because of hospital routines or perhaps prematurity can cause a delay in the normal mother-child attachment. While these facts must signify a psychological effect on a cesarean baby, the effect is not brought about by the delivery itself.

Physiologically, a cesarean delivery seems to have no real impact on a baby either at birth or in its future development. When a cesarean baby is well delivered and is not in distress, it cries just as promptly after delivery and has the same kind of Apgar score (measurement of a newborn's health) as any other baby. And the old cliché that cesarean infants are beautiful at birth is quite true, since their heads have not been molded by the trip through the birth canal.

Your baby will probably be born with more mucus than usual in the upper portions of its pulmonary tract—mucus that normally would have been squeezed out during birth—but this is no problem for a healthy infant. Most of it will be removed with a suction bulb in the delivery room and then in the nursery, and the rest will be coughed out easily.

A healthy cesarean baby emerges from your body looking just the same as any other baby, except for its nicely formed head. It is usually covered with cream-colored sticky vernix, amniotic fluid, blood, and perhaps meconium, the dark greenish contents of the bowel, and will require a thorough wipedown. Remember that the blood is from the incisions and not from the baby. When it is first born, the baby will be wrinkled and a little blue like other babies and will take a few minutes to "pink up," just as they do.

Simply because your baby arrived abdominally is no reason to believe it will be any less healthy and strong than it should be, assuming, of course, it is mature and there have been no difficulties either with the birth itself or with the pregnancy. Cesarean babies are not, simply because of the method of delivery, more fragile than other babies. Unfortunately, many women assume they are, partly because in many hospitals, even today, cesarean babies are still automatically deposited in the high-risk nursery for close supervision, because the mothers must recover from major surgery and do not feel well for a few days, and because in conservative hospitals the babies are frequently kept separated from their mothers immediately after birth.

But a healthy cesarean baby needn't be handled or treated any differently from a baby delivered vaginally, and more and more physicians and hospitals are recognizing that fact. As that recognition grows, more women will lose their fear that they have produced a baby who is in danger or somehow not quite right. Though *they* must recover from a perhaps traumatic surgical experience, the baby has had an easier time being born than it would otherwise have had and it is in no way damaged because of the route it has taken.

BABIES WITH PROBLEMS

Sometimes, of course, a cesarean baby is in some difficulty at birth. Most often, this is because it was already in some kind of jeopardy and that is why the surgery was performed in the first place. Fetal distress, maternal hemorrhage, acidosis, poor fetal metabolism, and some maternal diseases may all be reasons for any baby—cesarean or otherwise—to be depressed or ill upon arrival.

A cesarean baby, just like a baby delivered by the vaginal path, will sometimes be depressed because of medications given to you during labor before the decision to operate was made. Every drug you take, either for pain or for apprehension, may act as a respiratory depressant for your baby because it inevitably crosses over into the fetal blood supply. While a depressed baby is not what one would wish for, just remember that it will rapidly respond to respiratory assistance, which is available right there in the delivery room.

Very rarely, a newborn baby will not be in the best of health as a result of the cesarean delivery itself. If it is born this way because of disproportion between head and pelvis after a long labor that fails to progress adequately, the head may have become jammed into the pelvis and will require manipulation to get it out. Meanwhile, because of of the stimulation of air and movement, the baby may take a few breaths of amniotic fluid, blood, meconium, or whatever is present in the uterus, and this could have serious effects.

THE PREMATURE BABY

The most common reason babies born by cesarean section have problems is prematurity. *Prematurity is not caused by cesarean birth,* however, nor do RDS (respiratory distress syndrome) or other difficulties associated with early birth develop as a result of the method of delivery. They happen because the baby is delivered too soon, before it is ready to emerge into the light. Sometimes, when the unborn baby is in some kind of trouble, a cesarean must be performed whether or not the baby is ready if there is to be a chance it will survive at all. Occasionally, though, an error is made in scheduling a planned cesarean, resulting in a premature birth. To avoid such errors, it is essential that the best maturity tests available today—sonography combined with amniocentesis and L/S ratio or foam tests—are made before a delivery date is decided upon (see Chapter 5).

Meanwhile, be assured that having a premature baby does not necessarily mean the baby is in serious trouble. Many premies are healthy and vigorous; most others require some help, but are on their own in very short order.

Difficulties Because of Maternal Disease

Babies born of mothers with certain diseases, most commonly diabetes, may also have health problems. These problems are not caused by the delivery but by the disease that necessitated this kind of delivery. Diabetic mothers, unless they have remained in good control of their insulin balance throughout their pregnancies, often have infants that are larger than usual, with significant amounts of body fat and an excessive number of red blood cells. And these infants usually develop severe hypoglycemia (low blood sugar) in the first hours of life.

Women with chronic hypertension may have "dysmature" babies, which means they are quite mature but very small. By four or five months, however, they usually catch up with their peers.

Only rarely today is a baby born with Rh disease (erythroblastosis fetalis), but it can be the reason for a cesarean delivery. Rh babies may be severely anemic and jaundiced and may require exchange blood transfusions.

⊠ 5 ⊠

Tests for Fetal Maturity and Health

When you are going to have an elective planned cesarean birth, or there is a chance that a cesarean might be necessary, it is most important to time the delivery so that your baby is mature enough to survive nicely in the outside world. After all, the reason to have a cesarean at all is to produce a healthy baby.

If your doctor waits until the spontaneous onset of labor, then, in most cases, the baby is at term. Usually, however, a cesarean birth is planned for about two weeks before your due date. It may sound simple to figure out just when that due date is, but estimates are frequently wrong. That is why many cesarean babies are born prematurely, before their lungs are fully mature, before their livers can function fully, and before their tiny bodies can properly adjust to normal temperatures. As a result of prematurity, they may develop RDS (respiratory distress syndrome), jaundice, or other problems.

Not every woman has a twenty-eight-day menstrual cycle; not every woman ovulates on Day 14. And not every woman can accurately recall the date of her last menstrual period. Besides, though the average mean length of a pregnancy is 278 days, many pregnancies are longer. If the baby is scheduled to· be delivered two weeks before term, and the calculations are off by another ten days or two weeks, the baby could easily be delivered a month or more before the actual due date. The baby will be premature.

So it is not easy for an obstetrician to pinpoint with any accuracy when a baby is due. Nor should the doctor even try to pinpoint it, when a cesarean is planned, without the help of fairly sophisticated tests that are available almost everywhere in the country today.

Trying to estimate a baby's size by abdominal palpation—simply feeling by hand—is notoriously inaccurate, rather like trying to feel a penny through a pillow. And even if it were possible to estimate weight fairly well by feel, we know that weight does not necessarily equal maturity. A tiny four-pound infant may be physiologically mature, while a six-and-a-half-pound baby may be premature.

When it is decided to deliver the baby before the due date rather than wait for the onset of labor, it is essential that various maturity tests be made. There is no excuse for a baby delivered by elective repeat cesarean to be premature or to develop RDS as a result. The tools are available and the procedures are simple. Every woman who is going to have a planned cesarean should insist that the tests are made. If your hospital or doctor is unable to provide this kind of obstetrical care, it may be wise to go elsewhere, even if that means having to travel some distance to accomplish it. When cesareans are scheduled at the right times, babies have an excellent chance to be fully formed and prepared to live a healthy life.

No test is perfect, and no doctor can predict perfectly in every case, but the best way available at this moment to assist in scheduling a cesarean is to test the amniotic fluid for the baby's lung maturity.

Sometimes, when there is some confusion about the exact time a baby is due, physicians will purposely wait for labor to begin before performing a cesarean. This way, they know the baby is probably ready. But if you wait for labor to begin spontaneously, it's important that you are going to have the baby in a hospital where anesthesia coverage and a blood bank are ready and waiting so that the cesarean delivery can be performed promptly whenever you are ready.

TESTING FOR PULMONARY MATURITY

Let's assume your delivery is going to take place a short time before term. It is essential that the amniotic fluid surrounding the baby in the uterus is tested in order to know if the infant's lungs are mature. There are several ways of testing for this: the L/S ratio, the shake test, the foam test, the fluorescence polarization test (FP value), and finally the somewhat complex amniotic-fluid profile.

A number of researchers have found that a substance called surfactant must be present in the fetal lungs so that the pulmonary surfaces can permit oxygen to pass in and carbon dioxide to pass out of the lungs once the baby reaches the air. When there is not a sufficient amount of surfactant, the transfer of these gases will be inhibited, and the baby may develop RDS, the number one killer of prematurely born infants.

Surfactant consists of several free fatty acids. It has been found that, when the ratio of two of these substances is measured, it is related to the relative amounts of surfactant material being produced by the fetus: thus the lecithin/sphingomyelin ratio, or L/S ratio. In general, when this ratio is 2.0 or greater, the risk of significant RDS is very small.

Shake tests and foam tests also measure surfactant activity, and when properly performed, they are quick and accurate. Besides, they are available at all hours and in all hospitals since they do not require a laboratory or trained technicians.

Fluorescence polarization is yet another assay of surfactant material in the amniotic fluid. It has some advantages over the older L/S ratio, especially for complicated pregnancies.

The amniotic-fluid profile measures the individual phospholipid components of the amniotic fluid and is probably the most accurate predicter of pulmonary maturity available today.

First, Sonography

Sonography (or ultrasound, or B-scan) is harmless, painless, and noiseless. It is used to give an outline of the baby's body, particularly its head, and to show the location of both baby and placenta, as well as the largest pocket of amniotic fluid for sampling. It can also give a ball-park notion of the maturity of the baby by allowing the head to be measured.

In sonography, high-frequency, low-energy sound waves are passed through the abdominal and uterine cavities and create an instant "picture" of the baby's body on an electronic tube or screen. The principle is identical to the sonar used to measure the ocean's depth or to locate schools of fish.

Sonography is extremely important because, for amniocentesis (see page 52), the doctor must know exactly where the baby and the placenta are.

The Procedure

You are asked to lie on your back on a table with your legs straight, wearing only a bra and a hospital gown. To increase the conductivity of the sound waves, your abdomen is lightly oiled with mineral oil. Now an instrument that resembles a microphone is passed back and forth over your abdomen to produce the picture on the screen. As good views of the baby's head and body appear on the screen, the technician takes instant photographs of them. It is these pictures that provide the "map" for the amniocentesis.

A sonogram costs from $50 to $100 each time it is done.

Now, Amniocentesis

Amniocentesis is the withdrawing of a small amount of amniotic fluid for testing. Once the sonography has been completed, the amniocentesis must be done promptly before the baby decides to change its position.

The Procedure

First the fetal heart rate is recorded. The oil is removed and your abdomen is wiped with an antiseptic solution. Now, as you lie on your back, a thin needle is inserted through the abdominal and uterine walls into the amniotic sac. About 10 or 20 ccs of amniotic fluid is withdrawn (the baby won't miss it at all) and sent to the laboratory for testing. The fetal heart rate is checked again just to make sure everything is going well.

The amniocentesis, though the needle looks terrifyingly long, is no more uncomfortable than having blood drawn from your arm. Most women agree it really doesn't hurt at all. And it's quick—the whole procedure is over in about three minutes. If you are apprehensive, however, this is a good time to use the relaxation techniques you learned in your prepared-childbirth classes.

When amniocentesis is done in conjunction with sonography, it is almost 100 percent safe. The ability of the sonography to map out the location of baby and placenta eliminates the risk of hitting either of them with the needle. There is a tiny risk of triggering the onset of labor, but this usually happens only in women who are about ready to go into labor anyway.

An amniocentesis can cost anywhere from $75 to $150.

USING SONOGRAPHY AS A MATURITY TEST

Measurements of the fetal head, using the pictures produced by a sonogram, may help a physician decide if the baby is mature. They can be used only as an indication, however, since the baby's head does not grow appreciably during the last few weeks in the uterus.

USING X RAYS AS A MATURITY TEST

In earlier days, it was common practice to X-ray the abdomen late in pregnancy in order to judge fetal age by the appearance of the bones. Today we have much better and safer tests.

TESTING FOR CEPHALOPELVIC DISPROPORTION

When there is some uncertainty about whether the baby's head is going to be able to pass safely through your pelvis, your doctor may order an X-ray pelvimetry. This will produce an X-ray picture of your pelvic structure, allowing the internal passage to be measured. The amount of X radiation the baby receives from ordinary pelvimetry is almost inconsequential at this stage of your pregnancy.

Once the X rays have been made, sonography can be used to measure the diameter of the baby's head.

If the numbers don't match up nicely and it looks as though the baby will be too large to make it easily through your pelvis, then a cesarean may well be needed. Most obstetricians, however, allow a woman to have a trial of labor before performing a cesarean section for CPD, even though the measurements seem to indicate disproportion.

Testing for Intrauterine Health

When there is some question about whether the pregnancy is proceeding normally and the baby is growing as it should, you will be given certain tests that help the doctor to know how healthy the baby is. If you are going to have a cesarean birth because you have chronic hypertension or diabetes or chronic kidney disease, for example, which might affect the rate of growth of the baby or might necessitate an early delivery, your obstetrician will keep careful watch over the pregnancy from beginning to end.

There is no single test that gives an absolute indication of whether the baby is doing well or not. Each test is only a rough index; but, taken together, several of them can give the doctor a pretty good idea of the situation of the baby in the uterus.

The following tests are not part of the routine for every pregnant woman, cesarean birth or not, but are made only when there is reason to believe a problem may exist, usually because of some maternal disease.

Sonography

The same sound waves used to locate the exact position of a fetus in the uterus can also be used to show the rate at which the baby's head and other parts of the body are growing throughout the pregnancy. Normally, the head grows about a millimeter or so every week until about thirty-five weeks, when growth slows down. By taking sonograms every four or five weeks, starting *early* in the pregnancy, the rate of growth can be plotted.

Estriol Tests

Used together with an oxytocin challenge test (see page 55), tests for the level of estriol in either blood or urine will give a fairly good index of how the baby is doing inside the uterus. Estriol is an estrogen, a hormone, manufactured by both the fetus and the placenta. A drop in the estriol level is not, in itself, an indication that all is not well; it merely means that further investigation must be made. Certain drugs, for example, such as antibiotics and cortisone, may cause the level to fall.

If they are to have any significant meaning, estriol tests must be made two or three times a week. This can become very expensive, since the cost is about $25 to $35 per test.

OXYTOCIN CHALLENGE TESTS

In this test, oxytocin, a hormone, is injected into your bloodstream to stimulate contractions. During the contractions, the baby's heartbeat is recorded. Many obstetricians feel that this test is the most sensitive index of fetal health available today. It is usually done when there is a drop in estriol level.

As you lie on a bed, a fetal heart monitor is placed on your abdomen to record the fetal heart rate, as well as uterine contractions. For about half an hour, the heartbeat is carefully recorded. Then an intravenous is started in a vein in your arm and you are given enough oxytocin to stimulate three or four or five uterine contractions. The heart rate is again recorded.

If there is no significant change in the fetal heart rate before, during, and after the contractions, the baby is judged to have a good blood supply and to be in no obvious danger for at least another week. If, however, a significant change follows the contractions, then the result is a "positive OCT," and a decision must be made about when the baby should be delivered.

When the results are negative, but the physician is concerned about the progress of your pregnancy, further OCTs and estriol tests will be performed periodically.

The OCT isn't at all uncomfortable; the contractions produced by the hormone are so mild you hardly know you are having them. Nor is it risky in any way, except that it may set off real labor if you are close to term. If you are going to have a vaginal delivery anyway, you may merely have your baby sooner than you thought. If you are to have a cesarean, today may be the day.

OCTs are not normally taken until late in pregnancy, when it is possible for the baby to live if it is delivered. If for some reason, an OCT is performed much earlier in the pregnancy, it may trigger premature labor. In this case, there is some risk, but you must take that risk if the reason for making the test is pressing enough.

Each OCT costs about $50 and takes about an hour.

NON-STRESS TEST

For some indication of how a pregnancy is proceeding, you may simply be put in bed while the fetal heart rate is recorded for half an hour or an hour. The rate and beat pattern in response to the baby's movements will be a rough indication of fetal health and activity.

FETAL BREATHING/FETAL ACTIVITY SONOGRAPHIC TEST

With major advances being made in sonographic instruments and techniques, it's now possible to measure intra-uterine fetal activity quite accurately. Some experienced researchers believe that the rate of fetal respiratory chest movements are directly proportional to fetal health. Furthermore, rapid advances are underway to improve intrauterine health by changes in maternal activity and medication.

FETAL ACTIVITY DIARY

High-risk patients—those with some significant disease—may be asked to lie down at home for half an hour three times a day and simply record how many times the baby kicks. In about five days, a pattern of activity is established. If the pattern suddenly changes and the activity decreases, it may be a sign of some difficulty and requires investigation. Electronic means to record fetal activity more accurately are being developed and will soon be available in many medical centers.

•　　•　　•

While none of these tests gives THE ANSWER to the question of whether your baby is doing well inside your body, they do give some reasonable idea of what is happening, especially when the results of several of them are considered at once.

They are seldom done earlier than about twenty-eight or thirty weeks of pregnancy because a baby born before that time has little chance of survival. If there is good reason to believe there is trouble, the testing should begin after thirty or thirty-two weeks.

If, after the tests, there is real evidence that the baby is threatened, a decision must be made. Is the baby likely to be better off in the uterus, even though there are problems, or will it fare better delivered and in the high-risk nursery?

If the decision is made that the infant should be delivered *now,* labor may be induced if your body is ready. If it isn't, a cesarean section is in your immediate future.

❈ 6 ❈

Anesthesia

Probably one of your major concerns when you contemplate having a cesarean birth is the kind of anesthesia you will receive. Obviously, some anesthesia is required, but which is best, and will you have a choice of the one you will get?

You will have one of two types of anesthesia: a *general* (*inhalation*) *anesthesia,* which means you will be unconscious throughout the delivery, unaware of everything that is going on until you regain consciousness in the recovery room, the mother of a brand-new baby; or a *conduction (spinal or epidural) anesthesia,* which will numb you from your waist down but will allow you to be wide awake for the delivery.

Only very rarely are infiltration or local anesthesias used today for cesarean births. Though "locals" were once fairly common, they are now reserved only for very sick patients whose bodies cannot tolerate the stress of a systemic anesthesia (one that affects the whole body). Local anesthesia for cesarean sections, no matter how carefully it is injected, is never totally free of discomfort.

WHICH ANESTHESIA IS BEST?

There is no perfect anesthesia. Each has its advantages and disadvantages, its possible risks and side effects. But in the hands of competent anesthesiologists, a respected and important part of the childbirth team, all have become remarkably safe today. Indeed, this is one of the reasons why cesareans are so frequently chosen as the preferred method of delivering a baby when complications arise. Problems resulting from anesthesia have become *very rare,* just as rare as with any other kind of surgery.

The great majority of cesareans today are performed with a *spinal anesthesia,* though often the complication that makes the surgical birth necessary determines the kind of anesthesia to be used. Sometimes there is no chance for either the physician or you to make a choice. In a real emergency, when there is not a moment to waste, a *general anesthesia* is most often used because it is the quickest to administer and to take effect. With a general anesthesia, a baby can be delivered within about five to eight minutes.

Though a spinal doesn't take as long as an epidural, either to administer or to take effect, it still is not fast enough when there is a true emergency, such as severe fetal distress or maternal hemorrhage. Nor are either of these methods safe enough in these situations because they sometimes lower maternal blood pressure. If there is serious bleeding, lowered blood pressure can complicate the situation even more. And if the problem is severe fetal distress, which means the baby may not be getting enough oxygen, it may be better to go with a general anesthesia, which gives an easy means of increasing the concentration of oxygen to the mother and so to the baby.

When there is no severe emergency, the spinal is the

usual method of anesthesia. Spinals do not require exquisite skill to administer, and most obstetricians can even do the job themselves when an anesthesiologist isn't immediately available. Epidurals are another story. They are more difficult to administer properly than spinals and must be given only by anesthesiologists who have been specially trained in their use. Also, with an epidural, there is a greater time lapse between administering the anesthesia and its effect than with a spinal. This means there must be no immediate and pressing crisis requiring a very prompt delivery. On the other hand, epidurals do not produce the severe headaches that occasionally occur after a spinal.

HOW SAFE IS ANESTHESIA?

All three kinds of anesthesia have become *almost 100 percent safe today.* However, when problems do occur, they usually result from the use of a general, rather than from a regional, anesthesia. This is because it is easier for an anesthesiologist (or anesthetist) to commit a technical error in giving a general, and because a general requires more training and experience to administer well. Not only that, but the complex anesthesia machines can be misunderstood or misused.

The major complication that can result from general anesthesia—and it is very rare—happens when the mother breathes in gastrointestinal contents. It is for this reason that eating is prohibited before the delivery and that anesthesiologists now use an intratracheal tube (a tube inserted into your throat after you are asleep), rather than merely a mask, when giving a general.

There is also an element of risk—and again, it is very rare—involved with the conduction anesthesias. Not only is it possible that they may cause a drop in maternal blood pressure—and take longer to become effective—but it is sometimes difficult to administer them so that total anesthesia results. The "take rate" of spinal anesthesia when given by a competent anesthesiologist is about 95 percent; that of epidural anesthesia is about 92 to 93 percent. This means that occasionally an epidural anesthesia will be injected a second time in order to place it properly. Additional epidural anesthesia may be added if it's necessary. However, if a spinal anesthesia doesn't prove totally effective, a general must then be administered.

DOES ANESTHESIA REACH THE BABY?

There are physiological changes in both mother and baby when any anesthesia is used because any drug given to a pregnant woman eventually crosses the placenta. However, if the baby is delivered quickly after the anesthesia is given, this is no problem.

Different drugs cross the placenta into the fetal bloodstream at different rates, and are metabolized at varying rates as well. The effect on the baby of a drug given before or during a cesarean birth depends on the dosage, the route of administration, the particular metabolism of the mother, the health of the fetus, and the length of time between the administration of the drug and the delivery of the baby.

Recent studies have assessed neurological and behavioral responses of newborn babies during the first hours and days after birth. One study has shown that babies delivered with epidural anesthesia score significantly less well than infants born to mothers who have had natural childbirth. And it is possible to distinguish infants of mothers who have had epidural anesthesia from those born of mothers who have had general anesthesia. We do not know if any of these facts have any real significance in the long run; all we know is that they exist. But most experts agree that the modest amounts of anesthesias that normally get into the fetal bloodstream during a cesarean birth *do not* seem to have either a permanent or a detrimental effect.

As for the differences between the various kinds of anesthesias in their ability to cross over to the baby, it is quite clear that the general anesthesias (the inhalation agents) cross over the quickest. This does not mean they are necessarily dangerous for this reason. If babies born with a general anesthesia are delivered within ten or twelve minutes after the drug is given, plenty of time in almost every case, the babies won't suffer from respiratory depression, and will be born vigorous and active. If there is reason to suspect the delivery will take longer than ten minutes, then conduction anesthesia is advisable. This choice is often made, for example, for repeat cesareans when several previous abdominal births have made it very likely that there will be extensive scar tissue.

With a conduction anesthesia, the drug is transferred to the fetal bloodstream less quickly; this allows more time for a complicated delivery. With both spinal and epidural anesthesias, small amounts of the drug are transmitted to the baby's bloodstream, but under the usual circumstances, this involves very little risk.

Will You Have a Choice?

If your cesarean birth has not been planned in advance but becomes necessary because of the need to deliver the baby in a tremendous hurry, you will probably get a general anesthesia. Under these circumstances, no one is going to stop to consider your preferences and no one is going to take the time for a more complicated procedure. Everyone is going to be dashing about, getting you ready and the equipment prepared, and all the attention will be focused on delivering a healthy baby quickly. What is going on in your head will, unhappily, be virtually ignored. Though you may find this distressing, there is usually little time for a doctor to do anything more than say, "I'm sorry, but we must get your baby delivered fast."

But when a cesarean section is not a true emergency and there is no need for a mad rush to get the baby out, then you should be able to have your choice of anesthesias. Because of the trend in this country toward childbirth education and preparation, and an increasing desire by many women to have their babies as naturally and simply as possible, even those women who are having their babies abdominally are beginning to demand that they be allowed to remain awake and aware so they can witness their baby's arrival into the world.

And many women today want their husbands with them, too. (See Chapter 15 for a more extensive discussion.) Whenever and wherever this is allowed by the powers that be—the doctors and the hospitals—it is usually permitted only when the mother is awake for the delivery.

If you want to be awake, to witness the birthing experience, to partake of the first few moments of your child's life—if it is medically possible—there is no reason why you shouldn't have it your way.

Many women, though, don't want to be awake. Many prefer not to know what is going on; they want to go to sleep and wake up later when everything is all over. Sometimes the women who prefer a general anesthesia have been worn out by a long, hard labor and don't feel up to the experience. Sometimes they are fearful or squeamish, perhaps even afraid of what they will see and hear or what they will feel. Sometimes they would rather just skip the whole thing because it produces too much anxiety.

Occasionally, there are sound medical reasons why conduction anesthesia would not be appropriate or safe for you. As we've explained, when there is hemorrhaging or severe fetal distress, these anesthesias are not fast-acting enough and also have a tendency to cause a drop in blood pressure. Another reason can be obesity. If you are tremendously overweight, you will need much more anesthesia than the usual person and it may actually be impossible to administer an epidural or spinal.

And once in a while, when there is a serious infection that may have been precipitated by early rupture of your membranes, your physician may not want to take the chance of introducing those bacteria into the spinal canal.

General anesthesia is almost always available at every hospital, and sometimes it is the *only* anesthesia available. In many small institutions, the anesthesiologists (the physicians whose specialty is anesthesia) or the anesthetists (nurses trained to administer drugs) have not been trained to give conduction anesthesia. Sometimes it is the hospital's policy not to offer it. If your hospital does not offer it, your wishes to have it are quite academic—you can't.

And often, again in the smaller hospitals where there is no twenty-four-hour around-the-clock anesthesia staff (in 1971, only 8 percent of hospitals polled by the American College of Obstetrics and Gynecology had full-time anesthesia coverage for obstetrics), a specialist will be called in as needed. That specialist makes the decision about the anesthesia to be used. If you want a conduction type and he or she is able and willing to give it to you, consider yourself lucky and perhaps unusual. Many anesthesiologists feel most comfortable and familiar with general agents, especially if they do not specialize in obstetrics.

Even in the large hospitals, the anesthesiologist makes the final decision. This means that the person assigned to you may decide on a general for you, or perhaps for everyone. Your obstetrician, though he (she) may be happy to have your company during the birth, can be overruled. And, except in the most unusual circumstances, he does not choose the specialist he will be working with. There is a staff of anesthesiologists or anesthetists provided to the obstetrical department by the hospital, and the person assigned to obstetrics for that particular day is the one who will do the job.

In other words, neither your doctor nor you may be in a position to choose this specialist. And you will probably not even meet him/her until the night before the delivery, or perhaps not until that very morning.

If you are lucky, the anesthesiologist will ask you what kind of anesthesia you prefer and, if there is no overriding medical reason for choosing one over another, will give you what you want.

Though you can almost always shop around for the obstetrician you want to deliver your baby, it is almost impossible to shop around for an anesthesiologist. All you can do, in most circumstances, is hope your wishes will be considered. The main point to remember, though, is that a competent anesthesiologist is highly trained for one purpose only—to make you comfortable while your baby is being delivered.

WHAT CHOICE SHOULD YOU MAKE?

When you do have an opportunity to make a choice of the kind of anesthesia you will have for your cesarean birth, then you must examine your feelings closely. Do you really want to be conscious during the delivery? Will you feel you are participating in the birth, involved in it, even though the professionals are in control of what is actually happening? Is it very important to you that you see your baby at the first moment of its life? Or would you rather go to sleep and wake up when it's all over?

From a medical point of view, it doesn't really matter which you choose. Both general and conduction anesthesias, carefully administered, are very safe today. If there is a medical reason to choose one over the other, the professionals will decide.

Psychologically, however, there is a big difference between a birth under general anesthesia and one using a regional agent. The decision must depend on your own emotional makeup and responses. You must choose whatever is most comfortable for you. Both options are totally legitimate, and no woman should feel she must defend her decision.

For many women, early contact with their newborns just a few minutes after birth helps them tremendously to feel an emotional connection, an attachment, with their babies. It releases their mothering instincts and promotes an immediate bond. And being awake for the delivery makes them feel more in control of what is happening to them, less like a person whose destiny is being manipulated by others. Many women, and particularly cesarean mothers, are greatly concerned about their baby's health and appearance. Being awake for the birth lets them see and examine their new infants quickly, soothing their fears.

Most important, there is probably no experience more exhilarating than witnessing this moment of total creativity, this product of your own body.

For many other women, the desire to relax and rest, without fear or tension, especially after an arduous test of labor, is more important right now. They may not wish to witness everything or to be conscious of this "assault" on their bodies. They are quite willing to wait a few hours before starting their new lives as mothers.

Today, with so many women anxious to participate fully in childbirth, there is a tendency to put down the women who do not feel the same way, who do not wish to go along with the current trends in behavior. But the important thing is to do whatever suits you best, to make a free choice, to be comfortable with your decision. So talk it over—with yourself, your husband, your doctor, other women who have had cesareans—and come to your own conclusion.

IF IT'S IMPORTANT TO YOU TO BE AWAKE

If the kind of anesthesia you receive is very important to you, if you feel you definitely want to be awake for the delivery, then you must plan ahead if you can. When you know ahead of time that you are going to have a cesarean birth, or that it is a distinct possibility, be sure to discuss the anesthesia with your obstetrician early in your pregnancy or as soon as you know the cesarean is expected or suspected. If you wait until the last minute, it may be too late to influence the decision.

Ask the obstetrician about the kinds of anesthesia available at the hospitals in which he (she) delivers, ask his opinion on what kind would probably be appropriate for you, and question him closely about his feelings about having you awake for the event. If he obviously disapproves of conduction anesthesia for cesareans, or if his hospital doesn't provide it, perhaps you had best find another physician—and another hospital.

In many communities, unfortunately, you won't have many options. Sometimes there is no choice of another obstetrician, and often there is only one available hospital within many miles. In large cities, you can always find the doctor and the institution you are looking for. In New York City, for example, you can find ten good obstetricians within a radius of ten blocks, and, of course, there are many topnotch hospitals to choose from. In a rural, isolated area, or even in many small cities, you may have to go along with the traditional methods.

But let's assume that you have an obstetrician who is quite willing for you to have an epidural or a spinal, and that there are anesthesiologists in the hospital who are willing and able to administer it. If you alert your obstetrician early enough, he or she may be able to make sure that the appropriate person will be available on the day of your surgery. More and more anesthesiologists are being trained to give conduction anesthesia, and, because more women are demanding to be awake for their deliveries, more hospitals are providing it.

How General Anesthesia Works

With a general anesthesia, you will inhale a combination of gases, usually nitrous oxide and oxygen. At the same time, a curare-like muscle relaxant is added to your intravenous tube. First, you are given some oxygen by mask to increase your baby's oxygen supply just before the delivery. The anesthesiologist will probably tell you, "This is just a little oxygen for the baby. It isn't gas. Take some long, deep breaths." The mask may have a strange medicinal or musty smell from previous use or disinfectant, especially if it is made of rubber, but it is still dispensing only oxygen.

Then, before the anesthesia is given, you are put to sleep. You receive a dose of Pentothal or other barbiturate hypnotic through the intravenous tube in your arm, and in a few seconds you are sound asleep. (It is a common misconception that the Pentothal is the anesthesia. Pentothal does not anesthetize; it merely induces sleep. Its purpose is to facilitate the administration of the anesthesia.)

Now the anesthesiologist either places a mask over your nose and mouth or, more likely today, inserts an intratracheal tube down your throat, for the administration of the anesthetic gas. Then the muscle relaxant is added to the intravenous tube.

Once you are completely "under," the actual delivery of the baby takes only five to ten minutes. The repair of the incisions may consume another half hour or more.

Throughout the surgery, you continue to inhale the gas, remaining unconscious, and feeling absolutely nothing.

As soon as the anesthesia is discontinued, you are wheeled into the recovery room, where you gradually regain consciousness.

AFTER A GENERAL ANESTHESIA

The major side effect of a general anesthesia is the grogginess you feel for a good number of hours afterward. Another is amnesia. You will remember nothing of the delivery and little of the recovery room experience. You are sleepy for perhaps a day or two, or perhaps even longer.

Every person differs in her reaction to drugs. Some women function well as quickly as four hours after the anesthesia is discontinued; others are zonked out for a couple of days. Some women soak up anesthesia—especially if they are overweight. (This is because most anesthesias are fat-soluble and are readily absorbed and stored by the fat tissue.) Others take a long time to metabolize the drug, just as they might a sleeping pill or tranquilizer, because of their particular body chemistry.

Most people, however, excrete almost all of the anesthesia from their bodies within about twenty-four hours.

The return of sensation is rather sudden after a general anesthesia, and as you regain consciousness, you will immediately feel the pain from your abdominal surgery. This will require some pain medication, starting right there in the recovery room, and it will probably be continued every four hours or so for the first two or three days after the delivery.

CONDUCTION ANESTHESIAS
(SPINALS AND EPIDURALS)

Spinals and epidurals are fast becoming more and more common in hospitals where skilled anesthesiologists are available. With both a spinal and an epidural, anesthesia is produced through injections. of a synthetic derivative of Novocain into or around the spinal canal. These methods differ slightly, but importantly, from each other.

For a conduction anesthesia, you will be asked to lie on your left side on the operating table, curled as best you can manage into a fetal position with your back rounded, or you may be asked to sit up and bend forward. Your back is washed with an antiseptic solution and draped with sterile cloths, and then a local anesthetic agent is injected just to numb a small area where the spinal or epidural will be injected. You may feel a slight sting from the tiny needle, but that is probably the last discomfort you will feel until after the baby is born.

Now the anesthesia itself is given. The techniques are a little different for a spinal or epidural. First a tiny dose is injected to test for allergic reaction and the proper position of the needle, then the full dose. Your feet become warm and then tingly. The warmth moves up to your ankles, calves, thighs, and finally your abdomen. You feel a sensation of heaviness, which is strange but not uncomfortable, and then you feel nothing from about your waist down. With a spinal, you cannot move that part of your body.

When the anesthesia is fully effective, the delivery begins. Though you are awake, you are not able to watch the procedure because a curtain of drapes cuts off your view at shoulder level. You can see above and to the sides, and hear everything that goes on in the room as well.

Conduction anesthesias affect only the lower half of your body and have no effect on your mental acuity or your ability to stay awake. If you feel groggy or drowsy or dopey during the delivery, you have probably been given a preoperative drug, a sedative or tranquilizer. If you were in labor before the cesarean delivery, you may well have received drugs to relieve discomfort or anxiety, and these are continuing to have an effect.

Or sedatives may have been administered to you through the intravenous just before the surgery to keep you calm and collected. Some women can obviously benefit from sedation during a surgical birth if they are particularly anxious or frightened, but most women do not require it. If you do not want to be groggy during your delivery, discuss this subject with your obstetrician beforehand if it is possible. Make it very clear that you wish to be alert and awake, that you do not want a sedative or tranquilizer unless you specifically request it.

The major advantage of having a conduction anesthesia for your cesarean birth is that you partake of the birth experience, witness the arrival of your baby, see it, touch it, perhaps hold it. If you are having this kind of anesthesia for that reason, it makes no sense to be spaced out and sleepy, unless drugs are necessary for some valid cause. Nor does it make sense to take in more drugs that may cross over the placenta to your baby.

Even atropine, a drug usually given before surgery to reduce your production of respiratory mucus, is being used less and less today because it may have a slight effect on the fetal heart rate.

Once in a while, a cesarean patient needs sedation or some inhalation anesthesia during the repair of the incisions because of some discomfort. If this happens to you, you may find yourself feeling groggy then and in the recovery room.

ANTICIPATING A DROP IN BLOOD PRESSURE

Because conduction anesthesias can precipitate a lowering of your blood pressure, precautions are usually taken before the anesthesia is given. Your blood volume is expanded (this is called "preoperative loading") by giving you about a liter of an electrolyte solution intravenously.

This increases your total circulating volume of blood and compensates for the relaxation of the blood vessels that accompanies the anesthesia. You are always tilted slightly to your left during the delivery so that the pressure of the relaxed uterus will not fall directly on the main vein, the vena cava, that leads from the abdomen to the heart.

In the rare instances when these measures are not sufficient, you are given an adrenalin-like drug to maintain normal blood pressure.

SPINAL ANESTHESIA

When you have a spinal anesthesia, the anesthesiologist waits until the local anesthesia takes effect, and then carefully inserts a narrow-gauge needle between the third and fourth, or fourth and fifth, lumbar vertebrae, through the dura (the fibrous casing that surrounds the spinal cord and its fluid), and injects the anesthesia directly into the spinal fluid. This is not a complicated or difficult procedure. It is quick and simple, which is why it is the most common obstetrical anesthesia used in this country today.

A spinal takes effect rapidly, usually within three or four minutes. First you will have those odd feelings of warmth and tingling, and then total anesthesia and paralysis of your legs and abdomen. You are now turned onto your back, your abdomen is prepared and draped, your husband is admitted to the room if he is going to attend, and the delivery begins (see Chapter 8).

The average dose of spinal anesthesia lasts about an hour or an hour and a half, and this is plenty of time to deliver the baby and repair the incisions. There are some physicians who can do a cesarean "skin to skin" in twenty to thirty minutes; others routinely take an hour. Complicated cases obviously require more time.

Spinals, correctly administered, give very profound anesthesia and you feel nothing during the delivery, even though you are totally conscious. If, by some unusual chance, the spinal should happen to start to wear off before the surgery is completed, you will receive a second kind of anesthesia. Usually this is merely intravenous Demerol. If the Demerol does not provide sufficient coverage, you will probably receive a little general anesthesia by mask.

THE CHANCE OF A SPINAL HEADACHE

Somewhere between 1 and 2 percent of the people having spinal anesthesias develop very unpleasant "spinal headaches." These may last three or four days, though usually they last only about two.

Spinal headaches are caused by the escape of cerebral-spinal fluid from the hole that is made in the dura when the anesthesia is given (see page 72). When this fluid escapes, it lessens the fluid pressure on the brain and spinal cord and it may possibly react on the pain-sensitive structures within the skull—especially if the head is raised—thus causing a headache. Spinal headaches are not totally avoidable, even if you do lie flat on your back, never stirring, for the prescribed length of time. But with the tiny-gauge needles now being used they are becoming less common.

With a spinal, it is imperative that you lie flat on your back, without raising your head, for six to eight hours after the delivery. This takes the pressure off the tiny hole made by the needle in the dura, giving it a chance to seal over and heal, and reduces your chances of getting a headache.

Should you develop a spinal headache, you will receive pain medication and additional fluids, both intravenously and by mouth, to quickly increase your supply of cerebral-spinal fluid.

EPIDURAL ANESTHESIA

An epidural differs from a spinal in several important ways. A needle is inserted between the same vertebrae but only to a point just *outside* the dura (the fibrous casing that surrounds the spinal cord and its fluid). The needle is then replaced by a catheter tube. A test dose of anesthesia is injected through the catheter to make sure you will not have an allergic reaction and that the catheter is in the proper position. Then the full dose is given.

The long catheter tube is taped to your side or your shoulder, and you turn to lie on your back, tilted slightly higher to the left to take the pressure off the major abdominal blood vessels.

An epidural takes from ten to twenty minutes to take effect, with the warmth and numbness spreading slowly upward. You lose feeling in the lower half of your body, but you can still move. Meanwhile, the doctor and the delivery-room staff are preparing. If your husband is going to be with you, he is admitted now and sits near your head, behind the drapes.

Additional doses of the epidural anesthesia can easily be given if they are needed, simply by injecting more into the catheter. The average first dose lasts for about forty minutes.

Because epidurals are much slower to take effect than a general anesthesia or a spinal, they are never used when there is a real emergency. They do not always take effect with the first injection because they are more difficult to place properly, and they are not as profound as either of the other anesthesias.

With an epidural, you may feel some sensations during the delivery and the repair—feelings of tugging and pulling, or perhaps pressure on your upper abdomen when it is pressed down to help deliver the baby. This can rarely be called pain, but occasionally it can be quite uncomfortable.

You may feel a little dizzy or nauseous for a few moments, or feel the discomfort as a dull ache. Try using your prepared-childbirth relaxation techniques, or, if the discomfort becomes too much, you can let your doctor know you would like a little anesthesia by mask until it is all over or until more epidural anesthesia is given and has become effective. Most women, however, can cope with the odd sensations quite well and don't require help.

Epidurals do not cause headaches. You will be free to sit up in bed or raise your head without risking this side effect.

SPINALS VERSUS EPIDURALS

Spinals are much easier to administer than epidurals; they are much quicker and more profound. Epidurals require more skill on the part of the anesthesiologist because the anesthesia must be deposited in exactly the right place, and sometimes this requires more than one insertion. Not every anesthesiologist knows how to give epidurals, and not every anesthesiologist is comfortable giving them. On the other hand, even the obstetrician, with the help of a nurse, can give you a spinal if necessary.

So, then, why are epidurals given if spinals are easier, quicker, and more effective? The most important reason is to avoid the slight risk of a spinal headache, which can easily be the worst headache you have ever experienced or ever will in the future. Besides, additional doses can readily be given if they are needed, and the physiological changes in the body are somewhat less when an epidural is used. Less anesthetic agent is used; therefore less then circulates in your body to reach the baby.

AFTER THE DELIVERY

An important advantage of conduction, or regional, anesthesias is that the lack of sensation usually persists for about thirty to forty minutes after the delivery. This allows you to be undistracted by pain if you wish to hold your baby, talk to your husband, and adjust somewhat to your new phase of life. The spinal anesthesia almost always lasts that long, and an additional dollop of epidural can easily be given through the catheter to give you this added pain-free time.

In addition, the effects of a regional anesthesia are quickly dissipated and there is none of the grogginess that accompanies a general anesthesia. The feeling returns to your lower body gradually after conduction anesthesia, so that the pain of the incisions does not come on suddenly and fiercely as it usually does after a general anesthesia.

POSTOPERATIVE EFFECTS OF ANESTHESIA

When any anesthesia wears off, you feel the pain it was designed to disguise. At this time, you will need the help of pain medication to diminish the discomfort and allow you to rest. You may also feel nauseous, not only because of the anesthesia, but because of the activity in the abdomen and the displacement of internal organs. Though the nausea usually passes quickly, you may be given an anti-emetic drug along with the pain medication, as a precaution or a remedy.

No matter what kind of anesthesia you have had, the immediate effects disappear within four to eight hours after the delivery.

❈ 7 ❈

A Planned Birth:
The Preliminaries

While most first-time cesarean births come as a surprise, repeat cesareans are planned ahead, giving you plenty of time to find out exactly what is going to happen, perhaps even to help make some of the decisions. Planned abdominal births, though probably not the kind of delivery you'd pick as your number one choice, do not carry the same emotional impact as emergency cesareans because there is time to adjust to the reality of the situation.

Most scheduled cesarean deliveries are planned to occur just before your due date, although some obstetricians prefer that you go into labor just to be as sure as possible that your baby is mature enough to come into the world in good condition.

Almost invariably, cesarean sections are scheduled for early morning, around 7:30 or 8 A.M., which means you will probably have to check into the hospital the afternoon before. Not only will you have to be ready to go at that early hour, but several preparatory laboratory tests must be made before the surgery. Women who prefer to spend one more night at home with their families—especially when they have small children—often ask if these tests might not be made a day or two in advance so they may arrive at the hospital the morning of the delivery. This is an excellent idea and it can be done, but it isn't always possible to arrange. Most hospitals have set routines and are not very flexible.

There are some sensible reasons why you are asked to come the day before, aside from the laboratory tests. The medical staff assembled for the occasion does not want to be delayed if you are late arriving in the hospital. And, most important, it is easier for your doctor to be certain you do not eat or drink after a specified hour when you are safely in the hospital miles away from your refrigerator. Eating before anesthesia is dangerous.

So there you are in the hospital the afternoon before your cesarean birth. Extensive blood tests are usually made, more these days than ever before because of the threat of malpractice suits. These may include tests for uric acid, enzymes, blood sugar, electrolytes, hemoglobin, and so on. A urinalysis is always part of the testing procedure, and blood is always drawn to be cross-matched with one or two units of blood to be held ready in the blood bank on the small chance you will need it.

Most hospitals today do not take routine chest X rays of pregnant patients, but if a lung problem is suspected, an X ray may be needed.

After all the tests are completed, there is little for you to do for the rest of the day but rest and relax. You will be served a fairly bland dinner at an early hour, after which nothing else must pass your lips—not even water. It is essential that you eat nothing for eight to twelve hours before surgery.

THE ENEMA

At some time during the evening, or perhaps the next morning, you may be given an enema. To tell the truth, this is really an unnecessary custom; probably enemas need be given only to people who are constipated. If you've been having a regular daily bowel movement, and you would rather not have an enema, you can request that this procedure be skipped. Most doctors would probably agree to forgo it. If not, an enema is not the worst thing that ever happened, though it is certainly nobody's favorite experience.

PREPPING

Prepping is another custom that most women would like to avoid. This is the shaving of the abdomen and pubic area. Because the incision for cesarean section will extend to the pubic arch or just above it, and down into the pubic hair, some hair must always be removed. But a total prep is actually a prehistoric custom. There is no real reason, when you are to have a cesarean section, to have your entire labia shaved, just as, when you have a vaginal delivery, there is no real reason to have the upper pubic area shaved. If you object to a total prep, make your feelings known to your doctor before it happens, and perhaps you can avoid it.

Hair must be removed from the area of the surgery for some sound reasons. First, it is impossible to totally sterilize hair. Second, it gets in the way during the repair of the incision. So at least the top third of the pubic hair, along with any abdominal hair or even fuzz, must go.

Prepping happens the night before a planned delivery.

SLEEPING PILLS

Most obstetricians prescribe a sleeping pill for their cesarean patients. It probably isn't really necessary, unless you are especially nervous or apprehensive. But let your doctor prescribe one for you, and don't take it unless you need it. Don't worry about its effect on your baby—it will be completely metabolized before morning.

MEETING THE ANESTHESIOLOGIST

During the evening or perhaps very early in the morning, your anesthesiologist (or nurse-anesthetist) will come into your room to meet you. If you haven't already discussed the anesthesia you will get, do it now. Ask all the questions you have lurking in the corners of your mind, and make sure you get the answers. If there is no specific reason why a particular anesthesia must be used in your case, perhaps you'll be able to have your choice (see Chapter 6). At least make your preferences known.

CONSENT FORMS

Before your operation, you will be asked to sign a consent form for the surgery and perhaps, too, a form agreeing to a circumcision by the obstetrician, if your baby turns out to be a boy.

TALKING WITH YOUR OBSTETRICIAN

When you see your doctor the day before the delivery, make sure to find out exactly what's going to happen to you. This is your last chance to ask questions. Of course, it is best if you have gone over all these matters much earlier in your pregnancy, but, if not, now's your chance. Or perhaps you want to go over them again. If necessary, make a list of your questions so you won't forget any of them. Some doctors are not especially good at giving information, but if you are going to feel secure and satisfied, you must make your doctor give you full answers to everything you want to know. Don't accept the "I'm the expert, I'll take care of you, just don't you worry" approach.

If you are planning to have a spinal or epidural anesthesia because you want to be awake and alert during the delivery, tell the doctor that you do not want to be given any sedation or tranquilizers before the anesthesia or during the delivery. This is an important point and must be emphasized. Some physicians routinely give these drugs to every cesarean mother, and their effect is to make you relaxed, sleepy, and rather foggy. You won't need them unless you are extremely frightened and agitated. And you won't want them if your object is to be alert and conscious of everything that happens.

THE DAY OF DELIVERY

You will be awakened early on the morning of your baby's birth by a nurse who will put a thermometer into your mouth and take your temperature. The nurse will then take your blood pressure and check the baby's heartbeat. Though it is no longer general practice, you may be given a shot of a drug called atropine to dry your pulmonary secretions. It will make your mouth dry, too, but remember not to drink anything.

And now you are ready to have your baby.

8
The Delivery

In general, all cesarean births happen in basically the same way—whether they have been planned ahead or decided upon at the last minute because of a problem. The preparations are simply more leisurely for a planned delivery.

The order of events or the exact way procedures are carried out may differ slightly from doctor to doctor or hospital to hospital. This is the way it probably will be.

If you are going to have a general anesthesia, a catheter, a slim rubber tube, will now be inserted into your bladder. The catheter leads to a bag that will collect your urine. This is used because your bladder, which is located immediately in front of the uterus, must be kept empty and deflated during the delivery. When the catheter is inserted it may be a little uncomfortable for a moment or two, but it won't be painful. If you have learned prepared-childbirth relaxation techniques, you can use them now.

If you are going to have epidural or spinal anesthesia, you probably will not have the catheter inserted until after the induction of the anesthesia and so won't even feel a mild discomfort.

The catheter may be left in your bladder for a day or two after the birth, though this is not a good idea unless there are problems with the bladder. It is best to remove the catheter immediately to lessen the chance of infection. Occasionally a surgical patient (a cesarean mother or anyone else having abdominal surgery) has difficulty voiding after surgery, and some physicians like to leave the catheter in place just in case. If it is removed, however, it can always be put back in if needed.

To the Delivery Room: The Operation

When everything is ready, you will be moved to a rolling stretcher, wheeled to the delivery room, and shifted to the delivery table. In some large hospitals, there are special cesarean rooms; in smaller hospitals, you will probably go to the regular operating room.

An intravenous (IV) drip of dextrose and water (or other electrolyte solution) will be started in a blood vessel in one arm or hand to keep you hydrated during the delivery and for a day or two afterward, and to open a pathway for medication or blood should an emergency develop. The insertion of the IV needle may hurt a little, rather like an injection, but after it is in place it will be more of a nuisance than a pain. The needle is usually removed and replaced by a tiny flexible tube, secured by pieces of tape.

A blood pressure cuff will be wrapped around your other arm so that your pressure may be monitored. And perhaps you will be attached to an electrocardiogram. This is becoming a routine procedure in many hospitals. If you are, you will have tiny sticky pads placed on your shoulders and chest wall, and you will hear the beep, beep, beep of your heart. Don't let it make you nervous; it is merely a precaution.

Your abdomen and thighs will be thoroughly washed and painted with an antiseptic solution, then draped with multiple layers of cloths, leaving only a small area exposed. The drapes will be pulled up to form a screen at shoulder level so you won't be able to see below, just as they are for any surgical operation.

One of your arms will be strapped to an arm board, probably at right angles to your body. This is the one holding the IV tube. The other will probably be tucked under the drapes and maybe secured with a strap. This isn't done as some kind of medieval torture, but to keep you from moving your arm at an inopportune moment. If you find it offensive, ask if the strap may be omitted.

The order of these events will differ depending on whether you are to have a general or a conduction anesthesia. With a conduction anesthesia, you will be anesthetized first, before all of the above procedures in the delivery room take place.

WHAT YOU WILL SEE

Operating rooms are not designed for beauty, unfortunately, though some of the newer, special cesarean rooms are much less ominous-looking than the usual operating room. As you lie on the operating table, you will see the anesthesia machine near your head; a table spread with gleaming surgical instruments, sponges, gauze, cloths, and sterile drapes; a bassinette warmer in the corner, an oxygen tank, and several large overhead lights; nurses, anesthesiologist, obstetrician, and pediatrician.

GENERAL ANESTHESIA

If you are going to sleep through your delivery, this is almost all you will be aware of until you wake up in the recovery room. Before your anesthesia is administered (see Chapter 6), you will be prepped and draped, then given some oxygen by mask to increase your baby's supply just before the delivery. This is routine and does not mean there's trouble. The oxygen mask, especially if it is made of rubber, may smell strange, rather musty and medicinal. Take long deep breaths—all you are getting is pure oxygen.

As you are lying on your back, tilted slightly higher on your right side to take the pressure of the relaxed uterus off the major blood vessels, an injection of Pentothal or other rapidly acting barbiturate, along with a muscle relaxant, will be added to your intravenous. In just a couple of seconds, you will be sound asleep.

Now the anesthesiologist will give you the anesthesia—usually a combination of nitrous oxide and oxygen—by mask or through a tube inserted into your throat.

In five to ten minutes after the anesthesia has been administered, while you are totally relaxed and sound asleep, your baby will be delivered.

SPINAL OR EPIDURAL ANESTHESIA

For either a spinal or epidural (see Chapter 6), the anesthesiologist will ask you to turn over on your left side, rounding your back as much as you can. Occasionally the anesthesia will be administered while you are in a sitting position. Your back is washed and painted with antiseptic solution, then injected with a local anesthetic to numb a small area. This may sting just slightly.

If you are having a spinal, a small-gauge needle that you will not feel will now be placed directly into the space beneath the fibrous dura that surrounds the spinal cord, at about belt level. First you will receive a tiny dose of anesthesia to test for allergic reaction, then the full dose into the spinal fluid. Now you will turn onto your back again. In only a minute or two, your feet will start feeling very warm, then tingly. The feeling will travel up your legs and into your abdomen, and very quickly the whole lower half of your body will be numb. A spinal takes effect fast. You will be anesthetized and ready to go in three to four minutes.

A spinal usually "takes" on the first try, though occasionally the anesthesiologist will have to give a second or third injection. Before the obstetrician begins the delivery, he will test your sense of touch to be sure all sensation is numbed.

If you are having an epidural anesthesia, you will have a shot of local anesthesia, and then a needle will be inserted between two of the lumbar vertebrae to a point just *outside* the dura. Now a long, flexible catheter is inserted and the needle is removed. Sometimes more than one try is necessary to achieve complete anesthesia.

With the catheter tube taped to your side or shoulder, you turn onto your back, again with a slight tilt to your left. A test dose of anesthesia is injected by syringe into the tube, then a larger amount.

Now you must wait. An epidural takes anywhere from ten to twenty minutes to take effect. During this time, the lower half of your body slowly becomes warm and tingly and then completely numb.

Meanwhile, your abdomen will be washed and painted with an antiseptic, and the drapes will be arranged and the screen erected at shoulder level. The catheter will be inserted, the IV and electrocardiogram hooked up, and the blood pressure cuff wrapped around your arm. If your husband or someone else is going to be with you for the delivery, this is the time he is usually invited into the operating room.

Just before the delivery is to begin, you will receive

some oxygen by mask to give your baby a last-minute extra supply. Though the mask may smell medicinal, what you are getting is pure oxygen and not gas.

THE DELIVERY

When you are completely anesthetized, the delivery will begin. If you are awake, you won't be able to see what's going on, unless a mirror is suspended above the table for this purpose. And you won't be able to feel it, though you may, if you have an epidural anesthesia, notice some strange sensations of pulling and tugging and perhaps pressure. You will certainly hear all the sounds in the room—the clank of instruments, the voices of the medical team, the sucking of the suction tube, the shuffling of feet. If you haven't been sedated, you will be just as alert as you ever are. You can talk if you want to, but don't expect too much conversation from your obstetrician unless this is a doctor who likes to work and chat at the same time. Your husband, if he's there, and the anesthesiologist will usually be easier to communicate with.

Whether you are now asleep or awake, the surgical delivery is exactly the same. First the skin is incised, then the subcutaneous fat and the tendonous layer that covers the muscles of the lower abdominal wall.

The muscles are bluntly separated, and the peritoneum, the thin lining of the abdominal cavity, is opened, revealing the taut uterus beneath it. All this takes very little time.

If you are having a low transverse uterine incision, the bladder, which is attached to the lower front wall of the uterus, is freed and gently pushed down out of the way. This is usually not necessary for a classical incision. Now an incision, about six inches long, is made into the uterus itself. Your baby is ready to be born.

THE SKIN INCISION

Though two different incisions are made in your abdomen when you have a cesarean birth, the one you are probably most concerned about is the one that shows—the skin or abdominal incision. It may or may not parallel the one in your uterus.

From a cosmetic point of view, there is no question in anyone's mind that a "bikini" or Pfannenstiel skin incision is more attractive after it heals than a vertical incision. The bikini is a transverse cut from side to side across the lowest and narrowest part of your abdomen, at or just below the pubic hairline. When it heals and the hair grows back, the scar is usually almost invisible.

The vertical incision, on the other hand, is made in the midline of your abdomen, up and down from just below the navel to a point close to the pubic bone. It will probably heal beautifully, but it will always be somewhat visible. Occasionally, your vertical scar will be just a little off center. This is called a paramedian and is a little stronger than the midline scar.

The vertical skin incision is the quickest to make, and so it is often used when saving time is essential, when the major concern is to deliver your baby just as rapidly as possible. Sometimes, though, it's done because the obstetrician feels most comfortable doing it this way.

The skin incision will hurt for a few days after your delivery, then become sore and tender to the touch, and finally itchy as it begins to knit. But, in a few weeks, your abdominal wall will once again be healed and strong.

THE UTERINE INCISION

Though the incision in your skin is usually done bikini-style for cosmetic reasons, the incision into your uterus will probably depend on the obstetrical situation. A classical incision is made vertically through the main body of the uterus, while the low-flap incision, the most common kind, is made, usually transversely, across the lower segment of the uterus, which is narrower and thinner.

The classical is faster, so when there's a real emergency, this may well be the choice your doctor will make. It may also be chosen if your baby is particularly large, or is lying across the uterus in what is called a "transverse lie." Then the opening must be large, and the classical incision can always be extended up or down as far as necessary. The classical is sometimes the route chosen when there are dense adhesions or excessive scar tissue from previous cesareans, making access to the lower segment difficult.

The position of the placenta may also determine whether or not a classical incision is made. Occasionally the placenta implants itself in an unusual location. Instead of being attached to the upper portion of the uterus, it may be located over the lower part, blocking the baby's exit. This is called a placenta previa, and it can be an indication for a classical incision. This is especially true if the placenta is located on the front wall of the uterus. In this case, a classical incision is the safest choice because it eliminates the danger of cutting into the placenta during the delivery.

When there are no problems of time, size, or location, then the low-flap transverse uterine incision is almost invariably used today. There are many reasons why it is the preferred method. It becomes a much stronger scar than the classical, presents less danger of rupture in subsequent pregnancies, causes less blood loss because there are fewer blood vessels in this area, and has a tendency to produce considerably fewer postoperative adhesions.

The low-flap incision, however, takes more time to make and to repair afterward, and is limited in size by anatomic landmarks such as major blood vessels at each side of the uterus. At this level, the uterus can be extended laterally only a certain amount. The low-flap *vertical* incision is often used, therefore, as a compromise between a transverse and a classical. This, as its name tells you, is an incision made in the lower segment of the uterus, but it runs up and down. It is almost as safe from subsequent rupture as the transverse and can be extended into a classical if that becomes necessary. Usually it is ideal for a baby in a transverse lie because it provides a more roomy opening.

If you have had a previous cesarean section, then most physicians agree that you will have the same kind of incision you had before. In the first place, there is no point in being crisscrossed by scars, but more important, the abdominal and uterine walls can be weakened at the point where the two scars intersect.

You will probably end up with just one scar even if you have four or five cesareans. The doctor usually makes both the new internal and external incisions right through the old ones, excising out old scar tissue.

Most incisions heal promptly and neatly, though no one will ever see your internal scar again unless you have another baby by cesarean section. Most skin incisions heal with only the faintest visible line, though occasionally, if you have a tendency to form keloids (raised scars), a thicker scar will form. The eventual appearance of your scar will depend on your particular ability to heal and the resilience of your skin. In most cases, cesarean scars are not hard to live with.

THE BABY IS BORN

The membranes of the amniotic sac are ruptured, and the fluid pours out. The obstetrician reaches inside the uterus and gently lifts the baby out, while an assistant presses down on your upper abdomen. This is the moment when, with an epidural anesthesia, you may feel the pulling and tugging as well as a sensation of pressure. With a spinal, you probably will not notice these sensations because of the anesthesia's more profound effect.

And now, if you are awake, you will probably hear your infant's first cry, and in a couple of seconds you will know whether you have a boy or a girl.

The baby is held upside down for drainage of the respiratory tract, and its mouth and nose are carefully suctioned to remove amniotic fluid, blood, and mucus.

If the umbilical cord is long enough, your doctor may hold your newborn up for you to see before the cord is clamped and cut. Though there seems to be value, during a normal vaginal delivery, in delaying the clamping of the cord until it stops pulsating, this does not seem to be true during a cesarean delivery. And the obstetrician wants to repair your incisions promptly, as soon as the baby is handed over to the nurses and/or the pediatrician.

If you are awake, perhaps you will get a quick look at your baby now, or when all the routine procedures are completed in the delivery room. The infant will get an identification band around its wrist or ankle, and fingerprints or footprints will be taken. A pediatrician will make an initial examination, and the Apgar score (a measurement of the baby's health) will be taken at one minute and at five minutes after delivery. The baby will receive some oxygen if it is needed, and either an injection of penicillin or silver nitrate eye drops, depending on state law, will be given to protect the infant's eyes in case of infection.

(Note: If you are going to have the opportunity to spend the first hour or so with your baby in the delivery or recovery room, ask your physician *beforehand* to delay the eye drops until the baby goes to the nursery. "Eye contact" is thought to be an important part of the mother-child bonding process.)

The occasional baby who is born with problems will be

resuscitated in the delivery room and then taken immediately to the intensive-care nursery.

Now for the Repairs

While the baby is being cared for in its warmer, the doctor reaches into the uterus and manually removes the placenta. At this point, a dose of an oxytocic drug may be included in the IV solution for twelve to twenty-four hours. This acts to contract the uterus and control bleeding.

After taking a good look around at your ovaries and Fallopian tubes to check out their health, the doctor starts to close up all the openings that have been made. Though the delivery of your new baby has taken perhaps only ten minutes, the closing of the uterine and abdominal incisions takes much longer, maybe up to an hour or so.

First the incision into the uterus is closed with two or three rows of absorbable stitches, and the bladder is reattached in its normal place. The abdominal cavity is cleaned of fluid and clots, and the various layers of the abdomen are stitched back together again in their proper order. Finally, the incision in the skin is closed with catgut, nylon, or silk stitches, or perhaps metal skin clips, and covered by a tight gauze bandage.

When everything is back together again, you are wheeled off to the recovery room, where you will stay for a couple of hours before returning to your room on the maternity floor.

✖ 9 ✖

The Recovery Room

Your baby safely delivered and your incisions neatly repaired, you are now wheeled off to the recovery room, where you will stay for two or three hours of careful monitoring by specially trained nurses. In large hospitals with busy obstetrical departments, this room will be an obstetrical recovery room set up for brand-new mothers. In other hospitals, you may be taken to the general recovery room where all surgical patients, no matter whether they have had appendectomies, bowel resections, or a cesarean birth, are monitored together.

After a General Anesthesia

If you have had a general anesthesia, you will remain here until you are thoroughly awake, though later you may find you don't remember a thing about it, or perhaps have only a hazy recollection of having been there. The aftereffects of a general anesthesia vary from person to person. Some people are groggy and amnesic for a day, sometimes even longer, while others wake up quickly and are completely alert in only a few hours.

Occasionally, women complain that they have bad dreams or even hallucinations as they come out of the anesthesia; sometimes they can't recall why they are there or what is happening to them. This can be decidedly disturbing when it happens, but though it may not seem so, it passes quickly. An empathetic recovery-room nurse and the comforting presence of your husband, if he's allowed to stay with you, can help to provide the needed link to reality. Most people coming out of a general anesthesia feel as though they are simply waking up from a very deep sleep.

As you gain consciousness, you will feel the pain of the incision. The return of sensation is rather sudden after general anesthesia. It really will hurt, just as any wound does, though everyone's perception of pain is different. To help you cope with it before it becomes too severe, you will be given some pain medication by injection in the recovery room.

The most common pain medication used today is an opium derivative with the generic name of meperidine and the trade name of Demerol. Sometimes, however, morphine is preferred for patients who are particularly upset or frightened, because morphine, in addition to providing relief from pain, has a tranquilizing effect.

The medication will probably make you feel rather "spaced out," remote, distant. Some people report they feel as if they are floating. Others feel drunk. Some merely feel drowsy and rather dopey. For three or four hours after each injection of the medication, you will find the pain is nicely camouflaged and you will be able to get some sleep.

Pain medications, unfortunately, sometimes produce nausea. Added to the other possible reasons why you may feel nauseated now—the effects of the anesthesia, the disturbance of your abdominal organs, your relief from anxiety—this does not make for a happy time. It is not comfortable to retch or vomit after abdominal surgery. The nausea, however, that most commonly occurs during the first hour or two after the delivery, if it's going to occur at all, can be relieved by an anti-emetic drug. Sometimes this is routinely given as a preventive along with the pain medication. But if you have a tendency to feel nauseated easily, it would be wise to discuss it with your doctor before the delivery, so that he will be sure to leave suitable orders.

To help rid your system of the residue of a general anesthetic, the recovery-room nurse will ask you to take long, deep breaths and to cough lightly every few minutes. She will also insist that you move around in bed as much as you can.

REGAINING SENSATION AFTER A CONDUCTION ANESTHESIA

Spinal and epidural anesthesias wear off much more gradually than general anesthesia. You will arrive in the recovery room wide awake—unless you have been given a small amount of gas or sedative at the very end—and your perception of lower abdominal pain won't begin for a while. You may feel quite comfortable for perhaps twenty minutes or even an hour.

The area that was anesthetized first—the toes and feet—will be the first part of you to regain its feeling. After feeling in the toes comes back, sensation returns to the ankles, the knees, the thighs, and finally the abdomen. When this happens, you will begin to feel the pain of the incisions.

Now is when you will probably get your first injection of pain medication. There are a few doctors who use the epidural anesthesia as a pain medication for a day or two after the delivery. The epidural catheter is left in place and small doses of the anesthesia are added on a regular schedule. This works very well, but it is not commonly done because of the small risk of infection it involves and the fact that it prolongs the anesthesia and all of its effects, good and bad.

As the anesthesia wears off, the nurse will remind you to move your toes and then your legs just as soon as you can. It won't be easy at first because your muscles won't obey your brain, but the more you try, the sooner you'll regain full control of your movements again. The nurse will also instruct you to take long, deep breaths and to cough gently every few minutes.

With a spinal, you must be sure to lie perfectly flat on your back, without raising your head, while you are in the recovery room and for the rest of the day as well. No need to worry about that with an epidural.

Babies and Husbands in the Recovery Room

In a general recovery room, which may be a very busy place with a wide variety of intense problems, neither babies nor husbands may be welcome. The other patients may not wish to be disturbed, there may be concern for the baby in the presence of unavoidable bacteria, and the nurses, who may not be attuned to cesarean mothers and their needs, may insist on treating you like any other patient who has just had abdominal surgery. If your husband is allowed to enter the recovery room at all, it will probably be for only a brief stay.

But many hospitals, though they may bar fathers from the delivery room during a cesarean birth, permit them to come to the recovery room, especially when it is designed for obstetrical patients, and remain until you are taken to your room. If you can arrange this, do. It can be tremendously helpful.

And more and more hospitals will now make arrangements for your baby to be brought to you in the recovery room if you are in good enough condition to want it and the baby is in good health. If your conduction anesthesia has not worn off yet, there is no real reason why you can't hold your baby now and perhaps breast-feed, if that's what you'd like to do. With an IV in your arm and lying flat on your back, it may be cumbersome, but with your husband's or the nurse's help, you can surely cuddle a tiny baby for a little while.

If this is what you want to do, you must *ask* for it. Arrange for it before the delivery so that your doctor will make sure it happens.

HOSPITAL PROCEDURES

In the recovery room, the nurse will check you over about every fifteen minutes, taking your temperature, blood pressure, and respiration. She will examine your vaginal flow, your urinary output, and your surgical dressing. If your uterus is not contracting well, she will apply manual pressure to the uterus to push out any clots of blood that may be accumulating. This is not routinely done for cesarean mothers—nor should it be—because it does hurt badly. If you have learned relaxation breathing in your prepared-childbirth classes, use it now to make this discomfort easier.

When your body has become stabilized and all your vital signs are within normal limits, you will be transferred to your own hospital room, your home for the next five to seven days.

❈ 10 ❈

In the Hospital After
the Delivery

When the recovery-room staff decides that you are in stable condition after your cesarean birth, off you go to your own hospital room, where you are gently shifted onto your own bed. For the rest of that day, you will probably remain flat in bed (certainly if you have had spinal anesthesia), though some intrepid women manage to get up for a bathroom visit or a few steps around the room only a few hours later. The first day of a major abdominal operation is not known for its comfort. Your incision will hurt, and you will be rationing every move.

THE PAIN PROBLEM

Everyone's pain threshold is different and everyone's body reacts in a different way. Some women have great discomfort after the birth and others seem to move through the first couple of days with remarkable ease. There is usually much less pain after a repeat cesarean, because some of the nerves cut during the first birth never regenerate to be severed again. Mothers having their second, third, or fourth cesarean babies are often up and around much more quickly than they were the first time. But this is not a time to be a heroine or a martyr. You will receive pain medication as you need it, every three or four hours for the first few days. If you need it, don't fight it. Ask the nurses for it, if you need and want it; otherwise, they may assume you're quite comfortable without it. You will feel dopey and very sleepy a good part of the time, but sleep is good medicine. It is important to take the medication early enough each time to keep "on top" of the pain, so that not only will you feel more comfortable and in control of your body, but you will be better able to enjoy your newest family member as quickly as possible.

You do have the right to refuse the medication if you want to, if you feel you can get along without it, and some mothers can. Or you can ask that the medication be delayed for a while. Just remember that you have had surgery and that it is normal to feel pain. You are not a coward if you need help coping with it, and you would be most unusual if you did not. By the third or fourth day, you will need very little or maybe no pain medication at all, except an occasional aspirin or two.

TRANQUILIZERS, TOO

Sometimes tranquilizers are routinely prescribed for cesarean mothers along with the pain medication—especially after an unplanned delivery—to relieve anxiety. If you don't need any, there is no reason to have tranquilizers if you would prefer not to. Try to discuss this with your doctor beforehand. It is usually better to deal with your emotions right from the start, rather than put them off for a few days.

GETTING YOUR BABY

Most hospital staffs assume that a cesarean mother is going to be incapable of handling her baby very soon after the delivery—and sometimes through almost the entire hospital stay. But it all depends on the situation. Even if you are taking pain medication, you will be able to see and hold your baby when you are awake and not too uncomfortable. You probably won't feel well enough at least until about six or eight hours after the delivery, but then, unless the baby is in the intensive-care unit, you can ask that it be brought to you if you are not too sedated or too uncomfortable (see Chapter 11).

Just in case, tell your obstetrician *before* the delivery that you would like to see your baby that day. You may get the argument—from the doctor and later from the nursing staff—that cesarean babies must be carefully watched, that they tend to be "mucusy" and must be in the nursery, that you are not in good enough condition, that you might drop the baby or fall asleep while you're holding it.

But don't accept the argument. A normal, healthy baby, no matter how it is born, can certainly make the trip from the nursery to your room for a visit to its parents. Ask the doctor to leave orders for you to have your baby the same day, if you request it when the time comes. Of course, you should not be left alone with the infant if you are heavily medicated. If the baby's father cannot be there, a nurse must stay with you to be sure the baby is safe. Because the nurses' time is usually limited, an interested and involved father may be your best attendant.

Try to be realistic. If you are in a lot of pain or you are too sleepy to hold the baby, don't insist, though certainly the baby can be brought to you for a look and a cuddle. Or perhaps someone else will hold it at your bedside for you if you cannot manage it yourself. If four or five hours have passed since your last shot of medication and the drug has pretty much worn off, perhaps just a small dose now will be enough to keep you comfortable long enough to spend some time with your baby. You may even want to start nursing the baby, and that is possible, too (see Chapter 12). You needn't worry about the medication being passed on to the baby because the few drops of colostrum (see page 128) coming from your breasts now will not contain enough medication to harm the child.

MOVING AROUND AGAIN

That evening, or about eight hours after the delivery, you will be encouraged to sit up and perhaps even to stand or take a few steps. It won't feel good, but the sooner you do it, the more quickly your body will recover. Certainly by the next morning (or about twenty-four hours after the birth), you will get up out of bed. If this is a repeat cesarean delivery for you, you will probably find it easier to move around than it was the first time because you will have less pain.

Don't try to get up on your own. Wait for someone to help you. It will be uncomfortable, and you may even feel rather dizzy. By the way, you can get up with your IV and even the catheter still in place, though you can't travel very far.

EXERCISE IN BED

Between walks, and even before you get up for the first time, it is very important to have some exercise right there in bed. Wiggle your toes. Flex your calves. Push your feet against the end of the bed. Place a pillow under your knees and move your feet around in circles. Bend them up and down at the ankles.

Lie on your back, with one knee bent and the other

stretched out straight. Tighten your abdomen slightly. Now slide the bent leg out straight along the bottom sheet and back up again. Change legs.

Lie on your back with your knees bent and your feet flat on the bed. Now raise your head, hold it there for about thirty seconds, and then lower it.

You can even rock your pelvis from side to side—no more than is tolerably uncomfortable—and, lying propped up a little under your head and shoulders, your knees bent, reach forward with your arms and try to touch your knees. Don't go too far. Just a little stretch will do.

And try some cross-reaching. Lying on your back, your knees bent and feet flat, pull in your abdomen. Reach with your right arm across your body to the left side of the bed about waist level. Relax. Now reach across with your left arm to the right side of the bed. Relax.

BREATHING AND COUGHING EXERCISES

Every hour or so, or even more often, take a few very deep breaths. Hold your hands over your incision like a splint, and breathe in through your nose. Fill your lungs up with air, all the way down to the bottom, letting your abdomen rise gently. Hold it there for a few seconds. Now breathe out through your mouth until every bit of air is expelled, letting your abdomen fall again.

At first this is not a pleasant activity at all. But deep breathing will help to re-expand your lungs that are not being fully aerated because of the anesthesia and the discomfort you have been feeling. It will also help to rid your system of the residue of general anesthesia, help prevent postoperative pneumonitis, and reduce the amount of gas that accumulates in your intestines.

Coughing is another way to re-expand the lungs and get rid of excess mucus as well. Again, hold your hands over the incision and cough lightly. If you find this too hard at first, try huffing. Open your mouth, take a deep breath, then expel the air in quick, short huffs.

Using your hands as splints over the incision is also helpful when you sneeze or laugh or hiccup because it will inhibit painful involuntary movement of your abdominal muscles.

GETTING UP AND ABOUT

Once you've found you can get up and walk, you must be sure to get your exercise. Don't overdo it, but early ambulation will help get your gastrointestinal tract in full operation again and reduce the possibility of phlebitis, as well as pneumonia that once commonly plagued post-operative patients.

The best way to get out of bed those first few days is to roll the head of the bed all the way up so that you are sitting up straight. Now you won't need to use your abdominal muscles, but only your legs, to stand. If your bed operates manually, you will have to ask someone else to raise the bed for you. As the bed goes up, press back against it—you will feel more comfortable. Now bend your knees and slide your feet over the edge of the bed in one easy motion, pushing your torso up with your lower arm, until you are sitting up. Swing your feet for a little while before trying to stand up. Slowly put your weight on your feet, holding on to the side of the bed, ready to sit down promptly if you should feel the least bit faint. Slowly stand up, pushing up with your arms and using your legs for lift. Stay there for a minute before setting forth across the room.

Again—the first few times, call for assistance.

When you are standing, stand up straight, don't crouch over like an invalid. You will feel a pull on the incision, which may not feel good and may frighten you. But don't worry, you won't hurt the wound, and the discomfort will soon dissipate as you concentrate on getting from the bed to the door.

HELPFUL AIDS

There once was a time when incisions were bandaged and routinely covered by a "belly binder," a wide tape wound securely around the abdomen. Belly binders aren't used much any more, but they can give you a sense of comfort and support, especially if you have a particularly relaxed abdominal wall. Usually you will have only a tight gauze dressing, or perhaps merely a transparent plastic spray-on bandage. But if you think you would feel better with more support, ask your doctor if you might try a binder. Or you may find that a very lightweight stretchy girdle will give you that needed feeling of security.

If you don't already have them, ask someone to buy you a pair of elastic stockings. You may find they feel very good and they will help the restoration of circulation in your legs, especially if you have varicose veins.

GETTING NOURISHMENT

For twenty-four hours or perhaps thirty-six hours after the delivery, most cesarean mothers receive nothing by mouth, not even water except for an occasional sip. They are fed and hydrated, usually with a solution of dextrose and water perhaps supplemented with various electrolytes, through the intravenous tube. The IV will probably stay in your arm until you are back on some kind of real food, in about two days.

Because of the surgery plus the anesthesia, your gastrointestinal activity has been temporarily inhibited, and food will not move through your digestive system very quickly. But in about twenty-four hours, it will get going again and you will start to have small amounts of very bland and easily digested foods, probably broth and water, juices and gelatin. Even if you think you are starving, don't ask a visitor to bring you food. Your digestive system is not up to it yet and you may heartily regret it if you insist on surreptitiously downing a roast beef sandwich on rye or even some cookies or cake. Nor should you drink carbonated drinks, which will only add gas to your intestines, or coffee or tea, which may be irritating and act as a diuretic.

Gradually, more interesting foods will be added to your menu. Be patient. The speed at which this happens depends on your doctor and the state of your intestines. If you are really anxious to eat more, discuss it with your doctor but don't try it on your own.

Meanwhile, especially if you are going to breast-feed, drink as much of the acceptable fluids as you can. If water doesn't appeal to you, try ice chips or ask for additional broth and fruit juices.

URINATING ONCE MORE

If you still have the catheter in your bladder, you will notice that the nurse checks frequently to make sure you are producing urine and to measure the amount. If your catheter is out, she will measure your output in the bedpan, or may ask you to save your urine for measuring if you use a bedpan in the bathroom. The purpose is to monitor your kidney and bladder functions.

You may have some trouble urinating after the removal of the catheter. This is because of trauma to the bladder and urethra during the delivery or because your discomfort makes you unwilling to push enough to get the urine out. Until the pain subsides and the swelling and trauma are resolved so that you can do your own urinating, the catheter may have to go back in. A nuisance, but no tragedy.

AFTERPAINS

Every new mother, cesarean or otherwise, will have afterpains. Afterpains are the symptoms of a normally contracting uterus. They usually start perhaps twelve hours after the delivery and occur at random times for four or five days. They are similar to menstrual cramps, range from very mild to quite strong, and tend to be especially noticeable and strong if you are breast-feeding your baby or if you have been given oxytocin to stimulate the contractions after the delivery. They also tend to be more prominent, not with the first baby, but with subsequent deliveries. Cesarean mothers get the afterpains, not because of the surgical delivery, but as a normal consequence of childbirth. It is part of every woman's postpartum recovery process.

If you have learned prepared-childbirth relaxation techniques, you will find they can be helpful now.

THE FAMOUS GAS PAINS

After every abdominal operation, including a cesarean birth, you may be beset by sharp gas pains. The crisis of the gas pains usually comes on about the third post-delivery day. This is a normal physiological phenomenon, though a mighty uncomfortable one for most people. It occurs when the intestines, which have been paralyzed by the anesthesia and surgery, start getting back to work. Material previously present in the digestive tract has started to produce gas, distending the intestines. As the intestines become active and begin to move this material along, the accumulation of gas causes the pain.

Though gas pains can be extremely uncomfortable, they usually last for only a day or two and it is best to take no narcotics, the usual pain medications, for them. The medication may alleviate the discomfort, but it will only prolong the agony by slowing down the intestinal action again.

A few other things may help, however. Sometimes a rectal suppository or a small enema, occasionally a very mild cathartic, or a rectal tube—ordered by your doctor and administered by a nurse—will help get the gas out. If you have severe pain, be sure to let the nurses *and* the doctor know and some help will be on its way.

Physical activity stimulates gastrointestinal function, so, even though it may be uncomfortable, try to move around as much as you can. You can get out of bed now and you can walk, so do it even though it hurts. And as you lie in bed, do some serious deep breathing, holding your incision and moving your abdomen up and down, a few times every hour. Try lying on your left side with your knees pulled up.

Though gas pains can be distinctly unpleasant, just try to remember they won't last long and are an inevitable part of everyone's normal recovery.

SHOULDER PAINS

Some people, after abdominal surgery, find they have a sharp pain in one or both of their shoulders. This is the result of a diaphragm that has been irritated by air and blood collected beneath it. The nerve that supplies the diaphragm emerges from the spinal cord at the shoulder, which is why you will feel it there.

This discomfort is perfectly normal and will last only a few hours until the air and blood are reabsorbed.

CONSTIPATION

All cesarean mothers seem to become very anxious about constipation. You may not have your first bowel movement for a few days, and it's nothing to get excited about.

If you had an enema or a good bowel movement before the delivery, your lower colon was thoroughly cleaned out. Since then you have eaten nothing or very little, so there isn't very much to come out.

Unless you are having a lot of discomfort specifically because you are constipated, which is pretty rare, don't worry about it. Just drink lots of fluids to keep the stool soft.

If, by the fifth or sixth day, you haven't had a bowel movement, ask your doctor if you need a suppository, or an enema, or perhaps some milk of magnesia. Cathartics are not a good idea now because they can cause cramps, more gas pains, and perhaps a need to strain, which won't be comfortable.

VAGINAL DISCHARGE

Just as you would after an ordinary delivery, you will have some vaginal flow now. The uterus will continue to bleed a little from the raw surfaces where the placenta was attached to the uterine lining, and will produce a discharge until it is completely back to normal. It will go on for at least two or three weeks, and may last for as long as eight weeks and still remain well within the normal range. If you don't have any discharge, be *sure* to let your doctor know. This is a normal and important part of your recovery.

The flow will be bright red for the first three or four days, then it will gradually become paler, and finally, after about two or three weeks, it will turn yellowish white.

A sanitary pad, changed every few hours, will soak it up. Use the self-adhering kind under a pair of panties, so you won't need a sanitary belt. If you prefer a belt, place another small pad over your incision so it won't rub. Don't use tampons for at least four weeks, or until your cervix is completely closed. Even though you may not have labored, the cervix may have opened slightly. Until it is closed, there is always some concern about infection.

REMOVING THE STITCHES

If your skin stitches aren't the absorbable kind, they will have to be removed about the sixth or seventh day after the delivery. Women frequently become terribly anxious about the prospect of having the stitches taken out. While it is uncomfortable, it really isn't unbearably painful and it's all over in a minute or two. Knowing that probably won't help much, because this is a time when your tolerance for discomfort is very low, and the thought of having the sensitive, healing scar disturbed once more is not pleasant. You can use your prepared-childbirth breathing exercises now to good advantage.

Sometimes taking the dressing off is more painful than taking the sutures out, especially if the tape is over pubic hair that is now starting to grow back. Ask your doctor if you may start working on the tape yourself, so you can slowly get most of it picked off in advance.

SHOWERS AND BATHS

Until the stitches come out, you will have to settle for local washups; but after they are removed, the scar will be healed well enough for you to take a welcome shower. Baths are another story. Some physicians think baths are not advisable for a few weeks after childbirth because of the possibility of water washing into the uterus and causing an infection. This is a very remote possibility, but, just to be safe, it might be best to wait about two weeks before you soak in the tub. Consult your doctor.

TIME TO GO HOME

Finally the day comes, usually about the seventh or eighth post-delivery day, when you and your new baby can go home to start living in the real world. It is an exciting day, and a tiring one. Though you may be ready to leave right after breakfast, you probably won't make it through the door until about eleven or twelve in the morning, after all the hospital routines are completed.

Your bill will have to be settled through the cashier's office, and is usually taken care of by a member of your family. The baby must be fed, usually around 10 A.M., and this will take about a half hour or forty-five minutes. Then the nurse will help you dress the infant for the first time, and perhaps provide a blanket or a carrying case for the trip. Accompanied by a member of the hospital staff, you will walk or ride in a wheelchair to the outside door of the hospital.

When you get home, take to your bed for the rest of the day, doing only as much as you must. Now is the time to be coddled.

❈ 11 ❈

You and Your Baby

One of the most controversial and important features of a cesarean birth has always been the separation of mothers and babies immediately following the delivery. In most hospitals, cesarean babies are promptly taken off to the nursery as soon as they are born, and kept there for at least twenty-four hours and maybe longer before their mothers even get a chance to see them.

Meanwhile, the mothers, assumed to be too uncomfortable to be able to cope for even a few minutes with a newborn infant, are treated just like any other surgical patients: in other words, invalids.

But if you are a cesarean mother, you are *not* just like any other surgical patient. You have given birth to a baby, and the time you spend together with the baby soon after the delivery is tremendously important, right now and in the future.

On the other hand, you have had major surgery and will have to go through a period of some discomfort and inability to move freely, especially if this is your first cesarean delivery. You will simply not feel well enough to take over your baby's care immediately. You may even sleep through most of the first two days after the delivery.

Solving the problem is not always easy, especially since so much depends on the policies of the particular hospital you have chosen and the views of your obstetrician and the nurses assigned to the maternity floor. And much depends on you as well. You may feel you would rather spend time with your new baby a day or two later when you are feeling better, or you may want, no matter what, to see and hold the baby *now*. Studies have shown that "bonding," a close attachment between mother and infant, comes more easily when there is very early contact between them. But if, in your case, that is impossible, there is no need to despair. You can establish your relationship a little later. People, infants included, are remarkably adaptable.

When you have had a general anesthesia, you won't see your baby when it is born and you will probably be asleep or too groggy to see it—or remember it—for many hours afterward. You cannot control the grogginess through willpower, although some women think later they could have if only they had tried hard enough. The best approach is to go along with the feeling, to sleep and to rest until the anesthesia wears off.

A Good Chance to Hold Your Baby

When you have a spinal or an epidural anesthesia, you are awake for the delivery and will see the baby as soon as it is born. If you have discussed this with your obstetrician beforehand, and he understands how strongly you feel about it, you may be able to hold or at least touch the baby in the operating room (assuming, of course, there are no urgent medical problems that will cause the baby to be taken to the nursery very quickly). At the very least, you can watch the baby in its heated bassinette in the corner of the delivery room.

Once you have reached the recovery room, you will usually have perhaps a half hour or more of comfort before the anesthesia wears off. This is a perfect opportunity for you to make your first real acquaintance with your baby. There is usually no reason, except for hospital routine, why you cannot hold him (her), even nurse him, quite comfortably with a little help from a nurse or, even better, your husband. Immediately after birth is the "maternal sensitive period," named by Drs. Marshall H. Klaus and John H. Kennell, of Case Western Reserve University School of Medicine, because, according to their now-famous studies, this unique period in the first minutes and hours of life when there is mutual receptivity to one another is the time when lasting attachments between mother and infant can best be begun.

Hospitals often have policies prohibiting newborns in the recovery room. Sometimes this is because there is no separate recovery room for maternity patients and you will be placed together with people who have had any variety of surgical procedure, from appendectomies to colostomies to prostate operations. Here the nurses may not be especially attuned to the needs of new mothers or the care of newborn babies; there may be concern that the other patients will be disturbed by the presence of a baby; and there may be fear of the transfer of germs.

IS SPECIAL CARE NECESSARY?

Some hospitals have a rule, or at least a habit, that insists that the babies must be taken to the nursery, sometimes even the high-risk nursery in the case of cesarean babies, on the assumption that the infant may be in some sort of trouble. For years it has been assumed that cesarean babies are seriously different from those born in the usual manner, that somehow they require a great deal of nursing care. This is not true. A healthy baby is healthy no matter how it was born. While there may be minor differences of scientific interest between a baby born abruptly and a baby born through a prolonged birth process, these differences have no important significance—if indeed they do exist—if the infant is healthy. Nor do they affect any of its normal responses.

Special care is needed if the baby was delivered abdominally because of severe distress, if it has some illness, or if it is premature, but it is not needed by the vast majority of cesarean babies. Most are normal, vigorous babies, delivered surgically because of previous cesarean sections or because they would not fit neatly through the birth canal, and they can safely wait to go to the nursery until after they have met and spent time with their mothers.

LAY YOUR PLANS EARLY

If it is very important to you that you spend time with your baby immediately after its birth, then you must let your wishes be known. Tell your doctor before, during, and after the delivery that you want to have your baby as early as possible—in the recovery room if that can be arranged. In a large hospital where there is a resident staff, a pediatric resident can make an initial newborn evaluation of the baby in the delivery room; in a smaller hospital where there are no residents to do this, you may ask your pediatrician to come in to evaluate the baby. If the infant is found to be perfectly normal and healthy, it won't need to go to the nursery until after you have spent time together. Some private pediatricians are willing to make this special hospital visit because they believe strongly in the value of the immediate bonding period between mother and baby.

All is not lost if you cannot have this early contact; but if you can, it can give you a good headstart in your loving relationship with your new infant.

Unfortunately, most cesarean mothers do not see or hold their babies in the delivery room or the recovery room. And, more unfortunately, many do not see them for many hours or even several days afterward. Again, doctors and hospitals assume that you are going to be so knocked out by the anesthesia, so concerned with your own very real discomforts, that you are going to be incapable of cuddling a baby. They discount a woman's powerful maternal feelings, even in the face of pain. Add to this the common opinion of medical personnel that mothers of new babies, whether or not they have had children before, don't know anywhere near as much about themselves or their infants as the professionals do.

While this approach is the one you will find in most hospitals today, it is changing in many places. If you are in a hospital with rigid traditional policies, then you will have to try to have an exception made in your case—or go along with the rules. Even if you cannot hold your baby in the recovery room, tell your obstetrician before the delivery that you want to see your baby the same day as the delivery, if you are feeling up to it at that time. Then, if you are awake and able to tolerate your discomfort, remind the nurse that the doctor has given orders for the baby to be brought to you.

You—or your husband—may have to be insistent, but usually you can win out and you will get your baby if only for just a little while.

Don't hesitate to call your doctor and let him know if the baby is not then brought to you as often as you would like. Don't wait. The doctor can act as your advocate.

THE IMPORTANCE OF TOGETHERNESS: THE BONDING PROCESS

According to Drs. Klaus and Kennell, "the immediate postpartum period does have major importance in the development of a mother's bond to her child," and the more time you can arrange to spend with your baby immediately after its birth, the easier it will be to form a close and lasting attachment. Mothers who are separated from their babies have a harder time forming this attachment.

Many teams of researchers have investigated the formation of mother-child bonds in animals, and have found that animals whose offspring are taken away at birth often reject them, or at least have a much more difficult time accepting them again when they are reunited. Goats, for example, will not accept their own kids after the young have been removed at birth for more than an hour. If over an hour goes by without contact after a sheep gives birth, the sheep's attachment to her lamb is greatly weakened. With variations, the same is true for all other mammals.

Though the bonding process is much more complicated in human beings, we do know that there is something extremely important about the amount and quality of time you and your baby spend together *very* early in its life. Drs. Klaus and Kennell studied mothers who had many hours of early contact with their infants and compared them with mothers who had only the brief contacts afforded by the usual hospital routines (separation after birth and first contact twelve to twenty-four hours later for feeding, and so on). The effects were long-lasting and significant. The women who had the most early contact demonstrated more affection and provided more attention to their children weeks, months, and years later. Not only that, but early-contact infants had fewer infections, gained more weight, and had more success with breast-feeding.

During the first hour or so after birth, both you and

your baby are "mutually receptive" to each other. The baby is unusually alert and responsive, and you are in a state of heightened awareness and excitement if you have not been sedated. If you can be together at this time, communicating with one another, touching, exploring, looking, it can be much easier for you to feel connected—bonded—with your infant, to know that this baby is yours, that you care and love and will be responsive to its needs.

Not only the first hour after birth, but extended periods of time soon after that, can help to initiate and nourish the bonding, the feeling of connection with your baby. So if you cannot be with your baby immediately after the delivery, or even for the first day or two, try to make sure you can have sufficient time together after that. With time, patience, and long periods of contact, you can make up for the delays most cesarean mothers have to endure.

Breast-feeding often provides a way to be close and to make up for time lost, because it affords skin-to-skin body contact and a mutual dependence and mutual pleasure. For some cesarean mothers, it is a way to prove to themselves that they are truly the mothers of their new babies.

EASIER AFTER A PLANNED BIRTH

Cesarean mothers have an especially difficult time resisting separation from their new babies. Usually, during an unplanned first cesarean birth, there is no way you can make sure you and the baby will be together right after the delivery or even many hours later. Even if you can, the experience may not be as you would like it. You may well have had a general anesthesia, which puts you out of commission for a day or two; you may be totally exhausted after a long labor followed by an emergency cesarean; you may be frightened and upset, angry, bewildered, disoriented—all of these factors can affect your immediate feelings about your baby.

But if your delivery is planned ahead, it is possible in most instances to make arrangements with your doctor and the hospital to have reasonably early and satisfying contact.

Ask to touch the baby while you are on the delivery table. Ask to hold it after the surgery is finished. Ask to spend time together in the recovery room. Ask to have the baby in your room as soon as you feel you want it. Ask to have it frequently after that. Ask to give as many feedings as you would like, if you are bottle-feeding. Ask to have the baby at three-hour intervals, if you are breast-feeding.

In other words, try your best—using your obstetrician, your pediatrician, and your husband as advocates, if necessary—to have hospital rules bent when it is important to you. Simply being a cesarean parent should not keep you from your baby.

ROOMING-IN

In more and more hospitals today, rooming-in is an option available to maternity patients. This means that the baby lives in the very same room with you, and you, with a little help from the nurses, care for it yourself. While rooming-in is not a realistic possibility for most cesarean mothers for the first two or three or perhaps four days, it can certainly be accomplished after that, if it is what you want. At first it is a physical impossibility because you will not be able to get out of bed with ease, lift the baby yourself, or even change diapers without some help. Once you are more mobile, you will be quite able to manage, though you should not lift the baby just yet.

An alternate solution to the rooming-in problem is to have your husband in your room around-the-clock. He could have a cot near your bed and care for your baby until you are able to share the responsibility. A few progressive hospitals are permitting this, and more are considering such a policy.

Your decision about rooming-in must depend on how well you feel. If every movement hurts, if you cannot get out of bed with some ease, and if you don't feel like exerting yourself, you will probably want to wait until you get home before taking over the care of the baby. But if you can move with some comfort by, say, the fourth day, it wouldn't hurt to try it if you want to.

For most cesarean mothers, modified rooming-in turns out to be the best choice. This is the plan that gives you the chance to have the baby for part of the day, perhaps the daylight hours, but lets the nurses take over the rest of the time. You will get tired very quickly and you may be glad for the opportunity to sleep and rest without the responsibility of a newborn twenty-four hours a day. If you are breast-feeding, of course, you must have the infant brought to your room during the night at feeding times.

Having the baby in your room with you for long periods also gives the father time and opportunity to hold and care for the new addition to the family. The trend today is toward wide-open visiting hours for fathers, and if your baby is in your room, he will become much more at ease with it before you both go home than he would have after merely peering at it through the nursery windows.

Remember that lifting, even if it is only a tiny baby, is not advisable so soon after the birth. Your incision will have little tensile strength until about fifteen or sixteen days after the delivery, when the scar heals and becomes strong. This means someone else will have to pick up the baby and hand it to you. Ring for the nurse to do the job if no one else is around.

Caring for the baby is undoubtedly easiest if your husband can spend time with you in the hospital. He not only will get to know the infant but will give you the help you need now.

Sometimes, when rooming-in is an option at your hospital, it is available only when you have a private room. Because this obviously costs more money, it may be a factor in your decision. But if you have medical insurance coverage, and if you can move into a private room only on the day you wish to begin rooming-in, you may be able to manage the additional costs.

IF YOU ARE NOT ROOMING-IN

Most cesarean mothers decide to wait until they are home before taking over the care of the baby. Besides, most hospitals still do not offer rooming-in, especially to cesarean parents. But that should not mean that you need see your baby only a couple of times a day for twenty minutes or so. If you are breast-feeding, you will get the infant frequently (see Chapter 12), about every three or four hours, day and night. But if you are bottle-feeding, it is quite possible the nurses will want to do most of the feedings in the nursery. It is up to you to decide what you want to do, and you have a right to feed the baby yourself: every feeding or only some of them, during the day or both day and night. If you cannot manage to convince the nurses that you want to have your baby for feeding as often as you would like, have your doctor leave orders, or enlist the aid of your pediatrician.

Sometimes your new infant will be in the intensive-care nursery because it has some respiratory problem or other difficulty that requires medical treatment or at least close observation. If it cannot be brought to you in your room, then you must go to the nursery. As soon as you can get out of bed and feel up to it, ask to be helped into a wheelchair and wheel yourself down to the nursery. Here

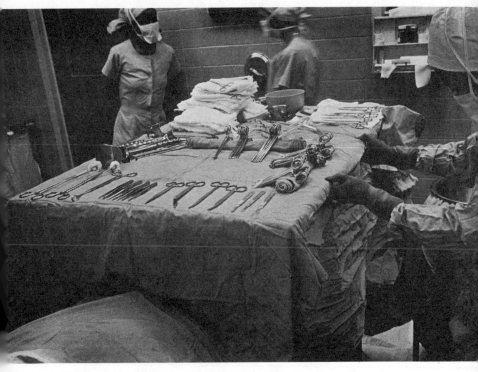

The delivery room: the staff prepares for your
cesarean birth.

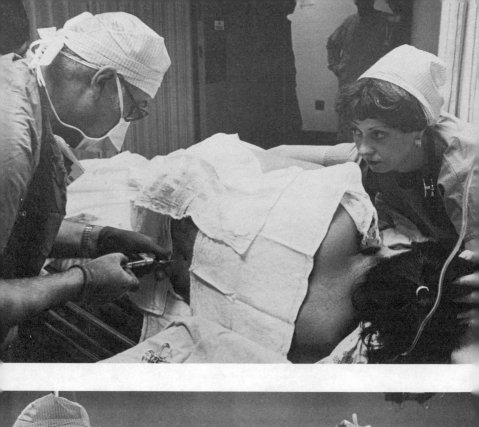
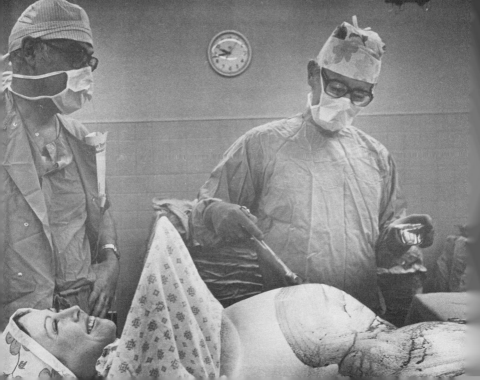

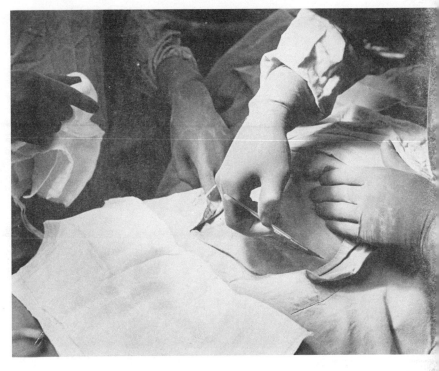

Obstetrician gets ready to make a "bikini" skin incision.

Opposite, top: So mother will be awake and aware, the anesthesiologist injects epidural anesthesia.

Opposite, bottom: The mother's abdomen is painted with antiseptic while the anesthesia takes effect.

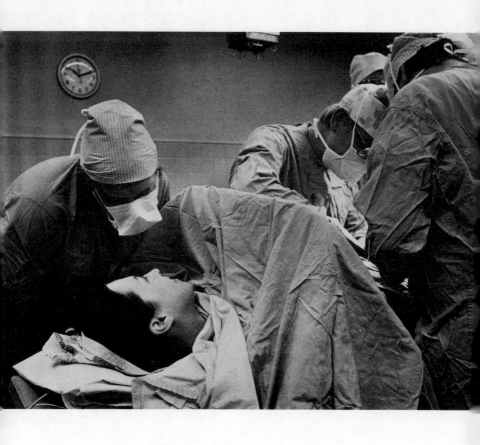

As the baby is delivered, husband and wife exchange
reassuring words.

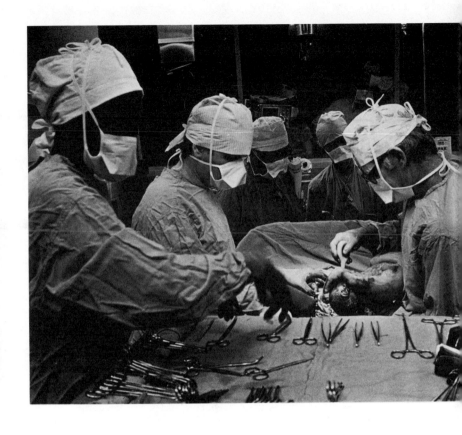

The new baby, in the first minute of life, is suctioned
and cleaned up neatly.

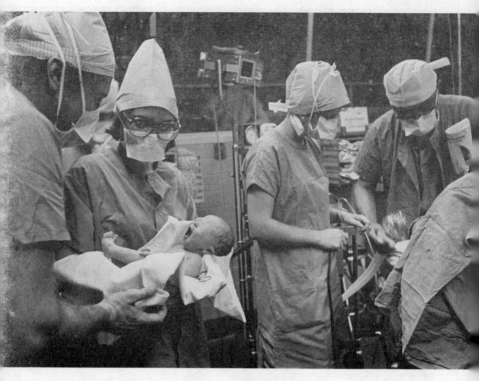

The new father gives his first-born child a big welcome.

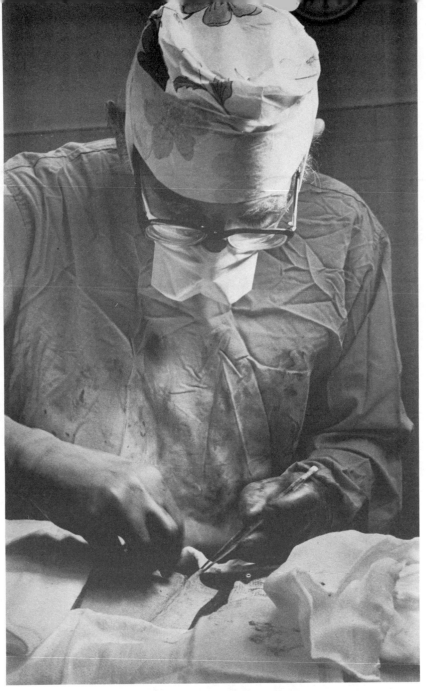

Repairing the incisions: sewing you up takes much longer than the delivery itself.

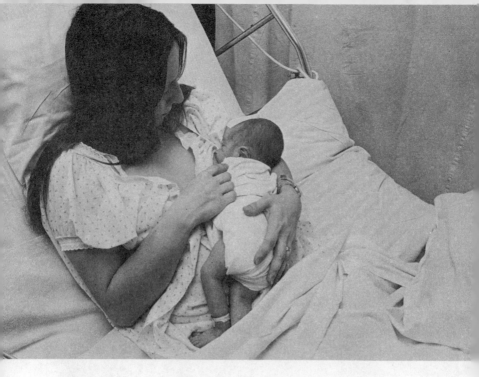

Breast-feeding a cesarean baby. You can do it successfully if you want.

Spending time with the baby helps you make that special "connection" right from the beginning.

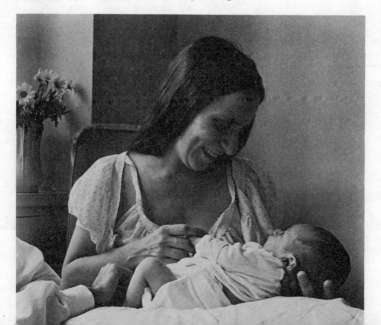

you can see the baby, touch and stroke him; and if the baby is there merely for observation, there's no reason why you cannot do the feeding yourself and spend time several times a day holding and cuddling him. You need that closeness, and so does your baby.

Again, you may have to make a fuss in order to accomplish this, though it is becoming standard practice in the more progressive hospitals. If you are told it is against the hospital's policies or contrary to the doctor's orders, get in touch with the doctor and tell him/her that you want to be with your baby. In most cases, the rigid rules will be bent.

VISITS WITH YOUR OTHER CHILDREN

When you have other small children at home, separation from them for such a long stretch of time can be difficult. Most hospitals prohibit young children from entering the maternity floor, though some of the family-centered institutions are beginning to change those rules. Though they usually do not allow small children in your room, they do provide a separate sibling visiting room.

Talking to your youngsters on the telephone helps a little, but not enough. One solution to the problem is to get special orders from your physician to be taken in a wheelchair to the hospital lobby, where you can visit with your children. Though they want to see the new baby, they are most concerned that Mommy is all right and will be coming home soon. Just the sight of you will reassure them.

A POINT TO REMEMBER

Meantime, remember that you have given birth to your own baby. It is not the property of the hospital, though the institution is responsible for giving it good care right now. Within reason—and that means if you are capable of holding a baby and that the baby is not sick—you have the right to have the baby with you a normal amount of time, whether or not you are a cesarean mother.

❊ 12 ❊

Feeding Your Baby

Just like any other new mother, you can decide to breast-feed or bottle-feed your baby. Many cesarean mothers are led to believe that breast-feeding won't work for them, but that is total nonsense (assuming, of course, there are no special problems in your particular case). Your production of milk has not been affected by the surgical delivery or the postoperative medications you have received, and you can breast-feed just as successfully as anyone else. You may, however, get off to a slower start and have a few more problems in the beginning for a couple of reasons: you may not feel very well for the first day or so, and you may be separated from your baby—for routine reasons or unique circumstances—longer than other mothers.

But it can be done if you don't panic, if you have patience and persistence, if you can elicit help from both your obstetrician and your pediatrician, and especially if the nursing staff in the hospital is cooperative and sympathetic. These are a lot of "ifs," but when your motivation is strong enough, and especially when you have decided *before* the birth that you want to breast-feed, you can usually do it. Many women have managed to breast-feed success-fully despite the subtle or open opposition they have encountered in hospitals, knowing that breast-feeding is the healthiest choice for their babies, besides being cheaper and much more convenient.

On the other hand, if you decide you do not want to nurse, bottle-feeding can be a totally rewarding experience for both of you.

In other words, make up your own mind whether to breast-feed or bottle-feed. The mere fact that you are a cesarean mother has no bearing on the method that you choose.

BOTTLE-FEEDING

If you are going to feed your baby formula, the infant will begin getting bottles in the newborn nursery and, when you are feeling up to it, will be brought to you dur-ing the day for regular feedings. You will probably find that raising the bed slightly at the head, and holding the baby close to you on one side, is the easiest way to feed for the first couple of days. You can lie on your back or turn over on your side. To burp the baby, simply turn him (her) over your shoulder or across your chest. Or you can lean the baby forward on your hand, with your thumb and forefinger holding his chin, the other three fingers support-ing his chest, and pat him gently on the back.

When you can sit up comfortably in bed or in a chair, a pillow placed over the incision will help protect it from the weight of the baby. Change arms from feeding to feed-ing, and take this opportunity to talk to your baby, cuddle him, kiss him, get acquainted. Taking care of yourself and your infant are your only jobs right now, so don't miss this chance to enjoy each other while you have plenty of time and no other responsibilities.

A big advantage to bottle-feeding is that someone else can feed the baby occasionally, and this may be a welcome help for the first week after you get home from the hospital. Fathers, especially, enjoy giving bottles, once they have gotten over their initial hesitation, and it gives them a chance to have their new child all to themselves even in the hospital. Actually, some fathers prefer their wives to bottle-feed rather than breast-feed so that they don't feel left out of the intimate relationship and can take an active part in nurturing the baby, too. If your husband can handle the nighttime feedings, at least for a few weeks, you will be able to get more sleep and so speed your recovery from the surgery.

With a first baby, almost every woman needs a little help in learning the best way to bottle-feed, and every hospital provides (or certainly should provide) some personalized instruction. When you have had surgery, you will need more help, and if it isn't forthcoming, ask for it. And if you want to give your baby all (or most) of the feedings yourself, let that fact be known. Many hospitals assume you won't want to be bothered—let them know you do. If necessary, insist that your obstetrician or pediatrician intercedes for you.

BREAST-FEEDING

There is a welcome trend today back to breast-feeding. Not only is mother's milk the most perfect food for an infant—providing immunity to some illnesses and causing fewer allergies—but it is, for many women, a tremendously rewarding experience. Giving your child something only you can provide is a very close, very private experience; it is also unbelievably convenient.

If breast-feeding is what you choose to do, it is a wise idea to let your doctor and the hospital staff know *before* the delivery. Alert your pediatrician, too. This way, they will be prepared to help you.

If you are awake for the delivery, and if you can get the cooperation of the doctor, ask to hold and nurse the baby right there on the delivery table, or in the recovery room. Aside from the exhilaration of being so close to your baby at a time when you are most receptive to each other (see Chapter 11) and of initiating the "bonding" between the two of you, early suckling stimulates uterine contractions by releasing oxytocin and hastens the shrinking of the uterus. It gets the whole process of lactation started a little earlier, and triggers the baby's suckling instinct.

The key to having this happen is good communication and an empathetic relationship with your obstetrician. Let the doctor know you really want to have your baby with you as soon as you possibly can. If it is understood—preferably before the delivery—that this is what you want, the physician can probably make it happen. Of course, if the baby is in any sort of trouble, however minor, and the prevailing opinion is that it should go promptly to the nursery for examination or treatment, then that consideration must come first. But most cesarean babies are perfectly normal and healthy and needn't be rushed off anywhere. They can be held in the warmer until they can be given to you for at least a few minutes before being taken to the nursery.

When you get the baby to breast-feed in the delivery room or recovery room, your conduction anesthesia is still effective for a short length of time, and you will be comfortable enough to hold him (her), look him over, love him. The nurse will help you. Even better, your husband, if he is there, will help you.

If you have had a general anesthesia, obviously you will not be able to nurse the baby in the delivery room, and you will be too groggy in the recovery room for more than perhaps a look and a cuddle, which you may or may not remember.

But, whatever the anesthesia, it is important to get your

baby as early as possible after the delivery if you are going to breast-feed. This does not mean you won't be able to do it if you are separated for a day or even two or three, but the earlier you get together, the easier it will be.

Keep in mind that, if you want to breast-feed, you can do it, cesarean birth or not. You may want to do it particularly strongly *because* you are a cesarean mother. Some women who feel they have "missed out" on the birth because of the surgery have an even more urgent desire to nurse because, they report, it makes them feel closer to their babies, more "motherly," more "normal." And if there has been a separation from the baby after the delivery, it allows them to achieve a quicker emotional connection.

It must be stressed: impress upon your obstetrician that you really want his help in getting your baby as quickly as possible. Be adamant. Do this before the delivery, and don't give up after it. More and more women, as they are becoming aware of their power as consumers, are choosing their doctors and hospitals on the basis of whether or not they are willing to provide what they want. And more and more doctors and hospitals are bending or totally changing their old traditional policies because they realize that, if they won't, women will find other doctors and hospitals who will go along with their wishes.

Usually, the chief barriers between cesarean mothers and breast-feeding appear to be the nurses. But you have to understand that nurses must follow the established policies of the hospital. Granted, some nurses are more rigid than others, but if, for example, your hospital's policy states that cesarean mothers are not to have their babies for the first twenty-four hours, the only way you can get around that is to have your obstetrician leave orders that you are to have your baby on demand or every three or four hours. Sometimes you will need to enlist the help of your pediatrician, as well, to put additional pressure on the establishment. And sometimes, of course, nothing will work because some medical policymakers cling to the idea that all cesarean babies require close observation in a nursery and that cesarean mothers want and need to be left alone for the first couple of days, undisturbed by their babies, to recover from the surgery.

But most women seem to feel better when their babies are with them. They can, if they really want to, overcome the very real difficulties, with some sympathetic help from the outside.

If you really feel poorly enough not to want to start feeding the baby so quickly, however, don't worry about it. You can begin a little later. You may even decide you would rather bottle-feed. The important thing is to do whatever suits you best, whatever makes you the most comfortable.

Don't be concerned if your baby is fed formula by bottle before you start breast-feeding. If you are persistent, the two of you will get along famously. If everything is normal, though, the baby won't need to be given milk in the nursery before you start nursing. In the first twelve hours of life, the breasts, even if suckled, produce little. Then for another twenty-four hours or so, only colostrum is secreted. This is a fluid that is high in protein and contains some antibodies that may protect the baby from infections, diarrhea, and other intestinal illnesses. It also stimulates the baby's digestive process.

For at least thirty-six hours after birth, you won't produce significant amounts of milk; and for about seventy-two hours, you won't make your maximum amount. The normal baby, in the meantime, will get along nicely on fluids—usually glucose and water—given by bottle in the nursery and on your colostrum. Because babies do not have a great fluid reserve, they become dehydrated easily and will need the additional water. But babies are not born hungry—by the time they need nourishment, your milk will come in.

DOES SEPARATION MATTER?

If you are separated from your new infant for a day or two after the delivery, for whatever reason, it will be a little more difficult to initiate breast-feeding than it would if you had started immediately after birth, only because the baby has become accustomed to a rubber nipple and an easy flow of water or milk. But this problem is usually quickly overcome.

A separation of longer than a couple of days can bring significant, though not insurmountable, problems. Unless the breasts are stimulated by suckling after the milk comes in, usually by the third day postpartum, lactation may decrease. So if your baby, because of prematurity or illness, is kept from you for a few days or a week after birth and you are determined to breast-feed, then you must express the breasts manually or by breast pump every four hours to keep up the milk production.

It is reasonable to expect a woman to do this for three or four or even five days if she is very anxious to feed her infant herself; to do it for a longer time than that is quite possible, but it requires such dedication and motivation that it is a very rare mother who manages it. But it, too, can be done. Many women manage beautifully.

Learning to express and pump your breasts requires application and patience. If you are lucky enough to be in a hospital where the nursing staff is knowledgeable and sympathetic, a nurse will show you how to do it, answer your questions, and bolster your determination. Perhaps your obstetrician can advise you as well. And if you haven't already purchased a book on breast-feeding, have someone pick up a copy for you so you may read and learn.

How Often Should You Breast-Feed?

Babies who get their nourishment from your body usually want to eat about every two to three hours, more often than bottle babies. If it is necessary, inform the nursing staff (and have your doctor back you up) that you want the baby brought to you every three hours or whenever he (she) is hungry.

The baby will come to your room for feedings during the day and, in some hospitals, during the night as well. In other hospitals, however, the baby won't be brought to you for night feedings for fear of disturbing the sleep of the non-nursing mothers. If this is the policy in your hospital, you will have to travel to the nursery at night. The first couple of days, you will probably have to be wheeled there. After that, you can walk the short distance down the hall yourself. Remember to remind the nurses to wake you at the specified intervals. Remind them again if they forget.

Can You Breast-Feed If You Are Taking Pain Medication?

You certainly can if the medication hasn't made you too groggy or sleepy to hold your baby. Even if the medication makes you sleepy, it will probably wear off enough to allow you to nurse in two hours or so after each injection. While you are on medication, of course, it is wise never to hold the baby when you are alone, just on the off chance that you may nod off.

Will the Medication Affect the Baby?

It is true that some of the narcotics in pain medications can be transmitted to the baby in breast milk. However—and this is important to remember—the average woman does not begin to lactate in any quantity until the third or fourth postpartum day. By this time, you no longer require much, if any, pain medication. You are usually able to get out of bed, move around, and eat real food, and the pain is not acute. The small amount of colostrum, perhaps a cc or so, that the baby gets at each feeding before that time will contain only an insignificant concentration of medication and will not have an adverse effect.

Even if you are still taking pain medication after the milk comes in, it is excreted fairly promptly. Even two hours after taking 50 mgs of Demerol or 6 mgs of morphine, which are the drugs most commonly used, very little is likely to be transmitted into your milk. It is not anywhere near enough to cause harm.

Usually by this time, if you need them, a couple of aspirins will make you comfortable enough for a feeding. If your pediatrician objects to breast-feeding while you are on regular pain medication, suggest that you try this. It is not a good idea to try to breast-feed when you are very uncomfortable, and most physicians agree that a tiny amount of pain medication or some aspirin-free pain reliever is preferable to a lack of success at the job.

GETTING IN POSITION

You will need to experiment to find the position that is most comfortable for you to nurse. According to the La Leche League, an organization that promotes breast-feeding, a good way to initiate suckling is to ask the nurse to lower the bed to an almost-flat position, leaving the side rails up. Now, using the side rails to hold on to, roll carefully to one side, asking the nurse to prop your back with pillows. Perhaps you would like a pillow, too, under your head, and under your uppermost knee. Now have the baby placed on its side, facing you, and you are ready to begin nursing.

If you would prefer lying on your back at first, have the baby placed on a pillow beside you, and, with your arm, press him (her) gently to your breast.

You can burp the baby lying down, too. Just roll him over onto your chest and rub his back.

To change to the other breast, place the baby on your chest, hold him securely, and roll over together. Let the nurse help you do it.

In a couple of days, when you are more comfortable, you may wish to nurse sitting up in a chair with a pillow on your lap to take the pressure off the incision.

BREAST-FEEDING MUST BE LEARNED

Breast-feeding is not truly instinctive and must be learned. You must teach yourself and the baby to nurse, so don't get concerned if you don't do it efficiently for a few days. There are several good books on the art of breast-feeding, as well as pamphlets distributed by La Leche and other organizations. If you take them to the hospital with you, you will find them helpful.

Even more helpful are private lessons, which are provided to new mothers by every good hospital today. Don't hesitate, if you think you are in need of help, to ask for it. Tension and anxiety are not what you are looking for, since emotional stress tends to inhibit milk production. The more relaxed you are, the better the whole process will work. If you are concerned that the feeding is not going well, ask the nursing supervisor to have someone give you more help, or discuss the problem with your obstetrician or pediatrician. If you don't speak up, no one will know you are having difficulties and you may become too discouraged to continue.

Remember that to build a good milk supply and to promote a quick postoperative recovery, it's important to eat high-quality, well-balanced meals with a sufficient number of calories and to get plenty of rest.

THE ADVANTAGE OF ROOMING-IN

When you breast-feed, it is especially helpful if your hospital has a rooming-in plan. You probably will not be able to have the baby with you constantly for the first two or three days, but after that, when you are able to get up with some ease, you may decide on this plan. Modified rooming-in usually works best for cesarean mothers. This means that the baby is with you during the day and in the nursery at night. During the nighttime hours, when the infant is residing in the nursery, you will go there or the baby will be brought to you for feedings.

AFTERPAINS DURING NURSING

Every woman who has delivered a child has some afterpains at random times for the first few days or longer, whether or not she has delivered by cesarean. These feel like cramps and are caused by the normal contracting of the uterus. Frequently, these afterpains are triggered by breast-feeding because of stimulated release of oxytocin. If you are especially bothered by them, a couple of aspirins taken about fifteen minutes before you feed the baby can help without affecting him at all.

※ 13 ※

Home Again

When you and your baby leave the hospital and get back home again, you are going to have to take everything slowly for a while. You have not only given birth to a baby, but you have also had a major abdominal operation. That doesn't mean you are an invalid, but it does mean you will have to take it fairly easy for at least a couple of weeks until you are feeling strong once more. If you do too much too quickly and become overfatigued, your recovery may be adversely affected, and it may take you even longer to get back to normal.

For the first week or so, don't put much pressure on your abdominal muscles. That means avoiding long climbs up steep stairs, as well as straining and heavy lifting. You will find yourself getting more fatigued than you ever thought you would be. You will be getting less continuous sleep at night because the baby will wake up frequently to be fed, and the physiological response to surgery means you will have a much lower physical reserve. Now it will take much more effort to do the simple things you used to do without a thought.

Taking it easy requires some planning—particularly if you've got other children at home. No doctor can tell you just how much time you should spend resting, and how much time you can be up and on your feet. You are going to have to judge how you feel and behave accordingly. But for at least the first week at home, you must keep your physical exertion to a minimum and spend a good part of each day resting.

HELP IS NEEDED

Household help after a cesarean is essential, and super-essential when you have other small children. Frequently these days, husbands take the week off to stay home and take over. If your husband can do this and is the kind of person who is able to cope with household chores and babies, that may be the perfect answer. It will not only take the burden off your shoulders, but give him a chance to get to know his new baby.

If this isn't the solution that works for you, perhaps your mother or mother-in-law, your sister, or a good friend will move in with you for a while. Housekeepers or even nurses, if you can afford them, are the answer for some women. In some communities, there is a homemaker service that will provide low-cost help. Whoever your helper is, he or she is the one who must do the cleaning, cook the meals, watch over the other children, and do the laundry and the shopping, as well as help you care for the baby. Don't feel guilty—you need to be coddled and you'll do a better job later on if you have had a smooth recovery. Meanwhile, you will have the time and the energy to enjoy your baby and to become thoroughly acquainted.

You will solve a lot of potential problems if you keep

the baby's crib or bassinette right next to your own bed for a few days. A new infant's needs are not great. The baby will sleep most of the time, will need only to be fed, cuddled, and changed. Bathing can wait till your helper has time.

If you are breast-feeding, caring for the infant is particularly easy. All you have to do is take the baby into bed with you for a meal. If you are bottle-feeding, it is helpful at first to use the prepared formulas, which don't even have to be heated but can be served at room temperature.

During the first week at home, the best way to pick up the baby is to have someone else hand him to you. If there's no one around to do that, try to place the bassinette at about waist level so that you may pick the baby up using only your arms. If you must bend down, don't bend at your back; instead, bend your knees, lower yourself to the level of the baby, and then straighten up again. This puts little pressure on the abdominal muscles.

Usually at the end of the first week at home, you will be capable of doing just about everything you did before—except for heavy lifting and too much of anything. Your incision will still feel tender and sore, but it will be almost completely healed. In another week after that, it will be really strong and you won't be able to harm it, no matter what you do. Sometimes, if you put significant strain on it, it can be very painful for a few moments. But don't worry, it doesn't mean you are coming apart at the seam. Of course, it is only sensible to be careful to increase your physical activities gradually and promptly stop if you become fatigued.

Though company is usually welcome and you'll want to show off the baby, keep the visitors at first to a minimum and only in short takes. If you explain that you tire easily and need your rest, even the most determined guest will get the idea and leave after a little while.

PAIN MEDICATION

Though you should not need it by this time, it is a good idea to take a prescription for a mild analgesic home from the hospital with you. It's comforting to have it just in case you have some lingering discomfort. But, if you're breast-feeding, avoid such medication. Trace amounts may show up in your breast milk and could possibly have some effect on the baby.

DIET

You may eat whatever you have always eaten, since your digestive system should be back to normal. But because you are not yet getting much exercise and are spending a lot of time resting, you won't require large meals at first, and you will probably feel best if you stay away from heavy foods. Try to get a good balanced diet, including plenty of fluids, milk, and high-protein foods to help your recovery along.

Just keep in mind, if you are breast-feeding, that whatever you put in your mouth gets into your milk, including medications, highly seasoned foods, and garlic. Ask your doctor if you should continue to take your prenatal vitamins. Supplementary iron is necessary only if you are anemic and your physician prescribes it.

DISCOMFORTS

As the days go on, you will feel less and less uncomfortable and much stronger. The scar will be sore and sensitive for a few weeks, though the area immediately around it may be numb. Some women find that placing a light dressing over the scar helps to prevent irritation from clothing rubbing against it.

Wear loose clothing for a while, preferably a dress or

housecoat that opens down the front. Snug pants, especially when they have fly-front zippers, can be uncomfortable and irritating to your scar.

Sometimes you will have freaky aches and pains in the area of the scar, lasting only a few minutes; sometimes it will feel as if it is twitching or pulling. These sensations come at random times, and you will feel them right at the incision or just to one side. Don't worry about them—they are perfectly normal signs of a healing wound. Later, the scar may become annoyingly itchy.

Scars heal differently for everyone. Don't be concerned if it becomes hard and lumpy for a while, or if it turns bright pink or purple. It will slowly soften and fade, getting finer and finer, and probably eventually turn white, much like a stretch mark. If you have a tendency to form keloids, or raised scars, this scar may heal that way, too.

INCISION PROBLEMS

Most incisions heal without incident, slowly and progressively. But once in a while, a wound infection will occur, and you should check your scar daily to be sure everything is going well. A small amount of clear fluid, barely enough to stain a dressing, is usually not a sign of infection and is nothing to worry about. But the discharge of any amount of brown fluid or material that has the appearance of pus—gray, green, or yellow—should be reported to your doctor promptly. And if you have any unusual pain localized to the incision area, with or without an area of redness, let the doctor know.

If you have developed a small superficial wound infection, the treatment is quite simple. Often moist heat is all you will need, but let your obstetrician make the decision after he (or she) examines you and perhaps takes bacterial cultures.

AFTERPAINS

These pains are rarely present by the time you go home from the hospital. They occur during the first few days postpartum, may be accentuated by breast-feeding, and tend to get more severe the more babies you have had.

CONSTIPATION

Because breast-feeding tends to be dehydrating for your body, you may have a minor problem with constipation if you have chosen this way to feed your baby. Make a point of drinking an increased amount of fluids. Milk, water, and fruit juices are good choices.

RETURN OF YOUR MENSTRUAL PERIODS

Your periods will probably not begin for at least six weeks after your delivery, and may not return on a regular schedule for up to three months. If you are breast-feeding, you may not start menstruating for five or six months, though you may have an occasional episode of vaginal bleeding. *Important:* remember that, though your periods may not return while you are breast-feeding the baby, this does not mean you may not ovulate. Breast-feeding is *not* a method of contraception!

During the first couple of weeks after the delivery, while your uterus is shrinking and the lining is slowly regenerating, you will probably have a bloody discharge. It will be a dark brownish yellowish substance that may not continue beyond three weeks or so, but for the average woman goes on for eight or nine weeks.

Often, women don't know whether or not they have had a true menstrual period. It doesn't really matter, unless you are planning to start birth-control pills. These should not be taken until after your first spontaneous period.

Though it may make you anxious to wait for your periods to begin again, there's no reason to get concerned until after about three months (if you are not breast-feeding). Beyond three months, it is worth mentioning to your doctor. The first thing the doctor will do is make sure you aren't pregnant; then he (she) will make sure there are no other difficulties.

SEX AFTER A CESAREAN BIRTH

Though most physicians are very conservative about the interval you should wait before having intercourse after a cesarean delivery, usually recommending six weeks, few couples wait that long. Intercourse isn't wise until your cervix is closed (if you've labored, there may have been significant dilating) because of the danger of infection, and that usually occurs within the first three or four weeks postpartum. If you never labored, it is certainly going to be closed three weeks after delivery. And at that point, it's safe to begin. None of this, however, precludes noncoital sex, which is medically acceptable at almost any time.

If your abdominal incision is comfortable and you no longer have any significant vaginal bleeding, there is no reason why you can't have intercourse *as long as* you use a good method of contraception. As a safety precaution against infection, make sure your husband washes carefully and uses a condom until your doctor provides you with another contraceptive.

Your incision may still be sensitive a month or so after the delivery, but you don't have to be concerned that you will harm it. It is now strong and secure. If it is uncomfortable, use positions where there won't be much pressure on the abdominal wall.

Until you have had your first menstrual period, when the hormonal mechanism gets going again, you will probably find that you don't lubricate sufficiently for comfortable intercourse. Because you are hypoestrogenic (which means you are still manufacturing far less estrogen than you did before, since your ovaries have not yet resumed their normal function), the vagina will not produce much mucus, and the vaginal lining may be somewhat thin and easily irritated. Lack of lubrication may also be a result of the emotional trauma of both the cesarean section and the process of childbirth. Use some kind of lubrication made especially for this purpose.

THE PSYCHOLOGICAL FACTORS

The psychological aspects of sex after childbirth, and especially after a cesarean birth, are often more inhibiting to new parents than the physical ones. To begin with, the baby may be sleeping in its bassinette right beside you and will make small noises and movements that are distracting. Even if the infant is in the next room or down the hall, you will hear sounds you never would have noticed before. Then, newborns wake up at unpredictable times. All new parents must adjust to having their own plans and desires go awry.

It's hard to enjoy sex if you are exhausted, and you may feel so fatigued after a long day that you won't be very interested in romance at night. After all, it takes time to recuperate after a surgical operation. Because your scar may still be sensitive, you will be concerned about hurting yourself, and your husband will sense your reluctance to be as freely sexual as you were before. And he may be twice as fearful as you are about hurting you, even though your doctor has assured you that it is perfectly safe. Sex, after all, is about 90 percent emotional and only 10 percent physical. It can be turned off by your head even though the body is quite capable of responding.

Add to these inhibiting factors a fear that many cesarean mothers have—the fear of having lost their attractiveness, their sex appeal, because they feel "damaged." They are afraid their mates will be repelled by their bodies, which are now, at least temporarily, stretched and scarred. Another psychological trauma often suffered by cesarean mothers is the feeling of having "failed" as women, that in some way they haven't functioned as normal healthy women do. Doctors have found that women who have delivered vaginally, but with the help of forceps, frequently feel the same way.

If you have these feelings of inadequacy, undesirability, or asexuality, you may find it hard to become aroused and enjoy sexual expression.

Scars are often, from a nonmedical point of view, not beautiful at first, even though they do fade eventually and often disappear almost completely. Just the same, you must realize that your emotional response to the way you have given birth is common among women who have delivered abdominally, and that it is quite acceptable to feel as you do. You are not abnormal. Talk to your doctor about it and discuss it with your mate. You will probably find that he doesn't consider it a turn-off, or that he won't for long, and that, with mutual understanding, you will soon be able to resume your sexual relationship without fear.

It's quite natural to feel cautious and tentative making love after such a major assault on your body. But if you take it slowly and patiently, if you both know each other's feelings about it and do not feel pressured to resume your old patterns before you really want to, you may discover a greater sharing and closeness than you ever experienced before.

THE NEED FOR CONTRACEPTION

Unless you want to become promptly pregnant, don't take a chance on having intercourse without contraception after childbirth. It's quite possible to conceive even three weeks postpartum, even though you are not yet menstruating again, and even if you are breast-feeding. Except under extraordinary conditions, it is not a good idea to follow one pregnancy with another so quickly. If you do, your uterus will not have the chance to return to normal, and your pelvic and abdominal muscles will not have become strong and resilient before they are once more stretched and strained.

Because most couples wait no longer than about four weeks after the delivery to resume sexual relations, you must make sure to see your doctor before that if it is possible. Do not take birth-control pills now, or use your old diaphragm. Until your doctor proclaims it safe to use your former method of contraception, use the condom as a safety measure. Don't take a chance with only foam or withdrawal.

If your preferred method of contraception is birth-control pills, wait until after you have had a normal menstrual period before you resume taking them so that you will be certain your uterus has gone back to its normal physiologic state. Of course, if you are breast-feeding, the pill must never be taken until after the baby is weaned.

If you wish to use a diaphragm, don't use your old one, but make sure you are refitted about four weeks postpartum. Even though you have had a cesarean and the baby has not come through the birth canal, you may not be the same size you were before. Not only that, but you must go back to your physician after another four weeks have passed to have the size checked again. The vagina may not return to its normal non-pregnant state for as long as two or three months.

As for the IUD, after a cesarean birth it is wise to wait for at least six to eight weeks before having one inserted, so that the uterus has totally involuted and returned to its normal size. Before then, the tissues are still soft and there is a chance of perforation. In the meantime, use a condom. Just be sure to use *something* every time.

POSTPARTUM EXERCISES

Your abdomen has been stretched during your pregnancy. Not only have you been carrying around, at the end, about twelve pounds of baby, cord, and amniotic fluid, but your body has been producing large amounts of estrogen and progesterone, which induce their own changes in the abdominal muscles. When you have had a cesarean birth, the muscles of the abdomen have been incised as well and now must heal. They will be tender and sore for a while, and so you will tend to use them as little as possible. It all adds up to a tummy that is not perfectly flat and firm. And unless you exercise, it never will be.

You will have no great need for "pelvic floor exercises," even if you have labored, because the baby has not pushed through the vagina. What you need are exercises that will tighten your abdominal wall.

Though some women become quite fanatic about it, there is little sense in starting tightening exercises before you are healed and pain-free. Wait until it doesn't hurt to move. Of course, whenever you start, you will feel a sensation of pulling and tautness in the area of the scar, but that will gradually diminish if you take it slowly.

Always start an exercise program slowly and work up to your maximum exertion very gradually. This advice is particularly essential to remember after surgery. It will be a matter of months before your abdomen is back in its optimum shape again. You will have to be patient, and remember, too, to do the exercises regularly. That means every day and over a long period of time. Most women start off after childbirth with a great flourish, then "forget" to do their exercises after about a week. If you really want good results, you must work at it.

Exercises will not harm your incision. By this time, it is as strong as it ever will be. If it hurts a little at first, that's fine. If it hurts a lot, stop and go back to less strenuous exercises. You may find that exercise will increase your vaginal discharge a little bit, but if the flow isn't heavy, it is nothing to be concerned about.

Here are a few abdomen-strengthening exercises that you can *begin* to do gradually about three weeks postpartum:

1. Lie on your back, one leg bent with foot flat on the floor, the other stretched straight out. Raise the straight leg off the floor a few inches, hold, then relax. Alternate legs. Don't try this with both legs at once—it puts too much strain on your lower back. Later, do the same exercise, but raise your head and shoulders off the floor at the same time as you raise one leg.

2. Lie on your back on the floor, knees bent. Hold your arms straight out toward your knees and curl your head and shoulders up off the floor as far as you can. Relax slowly. Later, try this with your hands behind your head.

3. Lie on the floor with your feet tucked under the edge of your bed or a heavy chair. Stretch your arms out straight in front of you and slowly sit up. Now slowly lie back down again, uncurling your back as you go. Later, when your abdomen is stronger, do this with your hands behind your head. Much later, eliminate the foot-tucking and do your situps without help.

4. Lie flat on the floor, feet wide apart, arms outstretched to the sides. Raise your head and chest as high as you can, and, at the same time, swing your left hand over to your right knee. Relax. Now do the same on the left side.

5. Stand with your feet apart. Clasp your hands at the

back of your neck. Point your hips straight ahead while you twist your upper torso from side to side.

6. Lie on your back, arms overhead, knees bent, and soles of the feet flat on the floor. Now pull in your abdomen and raise your hips off the floor. Hold for a few seconds and relax.

⌘ 14 ⌘

Psychological Aspects of
Cesarean Birth

Cesarean birth sometimes leaves scars, not just the scar you can see on your abdomen or the one hidden away on the wall of your uterus, but emotional scars that often last just as long and can hurt more. Though most cesarean parents probably have their babies without any serious or long-lasting psychological trauma, and settle down with their new family members almost as easily as they would have had they had the usual birth experience, some find that the experience of having a baby with the help of surgery can haunt them for a long time. It may affect the way they feel about themselves and the way they feel about their babies.

Any major surgery always and quite appropriately produces anxiety, especially when it is unexpected. A cesarean birth is not only major surgery, but also the birth of a baby in a manner that has usually not been anticipated or even allowed to creep into consciousness. As a result of this, it is frequently experienced as an attack on one's femininity, one's normality, and one's body. Add to that the difficulties many cesarean mothers encounter in their efforts to function as new mothers while they are physically very uncomfortable and immobilized, especially if they are treated like just any other patient who has had a surgical operation.

TODAY WOMEN ARE SPEAKING OUT

No scientific studies have yet been made of the psychological effects of a cesarean birth, and no hard data have yet been gathered, but cesarean parents have started speaking out, confronting their physicians about what has happened to them, gathering into groups designed to help them deal with their feelings and to educate themselves about their experiences. Certain feelings and responses seem to be extraordinarily common among these parents.

There is no way to determine the ratio of cesarean parents having good birth experiences to those having unsatisfactory birth experiences, especially since people with negative reactions tend to air them much more readily than those with positive ones. But it has become obvious that many women who have had abdominal births have strong and unhappy feelings about them, have been reluctant to talk about what they feel because they have been misunderstood, and find enormous relief when they discover that, far from being abnormal, their responses are remarkably similar to what other cesarean mothers experience.

THE IMPACT OF CESAREAN BIRTH

Becoming a new mother always requires emotional adjustments, but becoming a new cesarean mother adds its own special components simply because of the route the baby took coming into the world. Though one out of every five infants in the United States is born by cesarean section today, cesarean birth is not only "different" and, to some people, "unnatural," but also involves physical discomfort and a recovery period that does not accompany vaginal birth. A cesarean birth usually separates husband from wife, mother from infant, and all of them from taking a direct part in the birthing process.

The intensity of the emotional response to having a baby by cesarean section seems to depend on many diverse factors, including, of course, the self-image and sense of inner security you bring with you to the hospital, and the circumstances of the birth. The kind of physical care and emotional support you receive from your obstetrician and, often even more important, the nursing staff in the hospital, can make the difference between a positive birth experience and one whose negative overlay can have long-lasting psychological effects. The responses you get from your family, your friends, and the other women pushing baby carriages in the park affect your feelings about yourself and the birth experience. And, obviously, the way it happened is important.

A cesarean birth that has been planned ahead does not carry the same emotional impact as a surgical birth that comes as a surprise and is performed in haste and tension, leaving you no time to adjust, accept, or prepare—especially if it comes after many hours of active labor.

Most women who have "emergency" or unplanned cesarean births are totally unprepared for them and understand little except the fact that an operation is imperative in order "to save the baby." Usually they are terrified and confused over their transformation from a normal, healthy woman giving birth in the only way she ever dreamed of doing it to a surgical patient whose role as a new mother is overshadowed by the fact that she is having a major operation. Even women who have attended prepared-childbirth classes where the possibility of a cesarean birth may have been stressed have reported they never imagined it would happen to them.

Unless there is time for a detailed explanation and reassurances by an empathetic obstetrician or nurse, and often even when there is, most women who are precipitously thrust into this new situation feel enormous fear and shock. They fear for themselves and for their babies, for their husbands waiting outside, for their bodies, for the reactions of other people, and for their loss of control over what is happening to them.

Today, when so many couples prepare themselves to participate in what they plan to be a delightful, joyous, informed, dignified childbirth over which they have some control, the shock of having a cesarean birth can be especially devastating. No longer do they play principal roles in an exhilarating drama, no longer do they have a voice in making decisions about the birth of their baby, but, quite the contrary, the professionals take over. "When the doctor said, 'We're going to have to take the baby,' " one woman reports, "we both deflated so fast you could hear the whoosh."

Though the decision to perform a cesarean section may come as a relief if you have been going through a long and difficult labor with no promise of a quick delivery, most cesarean parents seem to feel, at the very least, disappointed. As one woman said, "Yes, I know I have a beautiful normal, healthy baby, but something is missing. I wanted to have this baby myself, just like everyone else. I wanted to have Jim there helping me and we'd do it together. Why did this have to happen to me?" She and her husband had had big plans, and the big plans didn't work out. They felt cheated out of an experience they desperately wanted.

FEELINGS OF ANGER

Anger is another response common among cesarean mothers—anger at yourself for not performing as you wanted to, anger at being put out of commission by the surgery. You may resent your baby for being too big, for not turning around in the right direction, for causing you all this trouble. Some cesarean mothers turn their anger on their doctors who "assaulted" their bodies, or on their husbands who wanted this baby and don't seem to understand how they feel or what they are going through.

FEELINGS OF FAILURE

It is certainly not uncommon for a cesarean mother to feel tremendous guilt because she has given birth abdominally, as if she had done something wrong or had not passed the test. She may blame herself for many things— not practicing her exercises, gaining too much weight, accepting medication during labor, not trying "hard enough," not resting enough. She may even blame herself, as one woman did, for feeling so good during her pregnancy that she didn't pay attention to the "little signs of trouble" she was sure she should have spotted.

If she feels guilty, she feels inadequate, too, and she is not unusual among cesarean mothers. She thinks that somehow she has failed, she "didn't do it right," she wasn't up to the job of having a baby the "normal" way. Many women have the feeling that they are "less of a woman," "unfeminine," "unwhole." Some feel disfigured, and others are sure they will no longer be attractive and desirable to men, including their husbands.

It is not possible to describe with any justice the myriad of feelings fleetingly or lastingly shared by most cesarean mothers after an unexpected abdominal birth—only they can put adequate words to what they have experienced. At the end of this chapter, we will let a few of them speak for themselves.

FATHERS REACT, TOO

A cesarean birth may well be a difficult time for the baby's father, too. If he had enthusiastically planned to share the birth experience, he will be intensely disappointed. Not only has he not participated, but he has been rejected, left behind. Even a father who hasn't prepared himself to be a participating member of the team—and most fathers do not—has special fears of this kind of birth. Though he may feel greatly relieved that the doctor has decided "to do something" about a labor that isn't going well, he is frightened. Will she live? Will the baby live? Will the baby be normal? What is going on? Why doesn't anyone tell me what is happening? Fathers frequently receive no information about their wives or babies for long periods of time after leaving them before the delivery.

He may feel responsible for his wife being in a condition that causes her to be cut open in order to have his baby. He may experience terrible guilt, and determine that he is never going to get her pregnant again if this is the result. Because of the fear of future pregnancy, some men become wary of sexual relations with their wives even with adequate contraceptive protection.

Unfortunately, some men join their wives in feeling the wife has failed in some way. And others cannot comprehend the disappointment, the sense of having missed out on an experience other women have. The baby is born, it is healthy, his wife will soon feel fine, and, as one man said, "What's the big deal?"

The inappropriate responses of family and friends may not be helpful. A woman who is depressed, who feels guilty, inadequate, angry, and who has a big pain in her belly, isn't cheered up by hearing, "But the only thing that matters is you've got a beautiful baby." She knows that, but needs understanding, help with her feelings, relief from the guilt of feeling them, as well as sympathetic physical attention.

Nor does it cheer her to hear her friends and hospital mates tell her their experiences having their babies the way she wanted to have hers. Or being told, "You're lucky, you did it the easy way." To her, it wasn't easy, nor does she feel lucky. One woman's hospital roommate told her she had to be biologically inferior and gave her a detailed description of her own husband-coached childbirth. A father-in-law walked into another woman's room and said, presumably as a joke, "Well, you flunked."

RELATING TO YOUR BABY

Adding to the psychological burdens of new motherhood, a cesarean mother sometimes has some difficulty relating quickly to her infant because of her confused feelings and the physical realities of a surgical delivery. In addition, her baby may be routinely placed in the intensive-care nursery simply because it arrived by cesarean or because it was delivered this way because it was already in some trouble. In many hospitals it is assumed as well that cesarean mothers are too concerned with their own physical conditions to be interested in spending much time with their new babies the first day or two or even three. Nor is rooming-in usually a possibility. For all these reasons, it is not uncommon to be delayed in forming a close connection with the baby. All that can be made up in time, given enough motivation and support, but, in the meantime, it can add another reason to feel guilty and unworthy as well as to assume the baby is "delicate" and sickly and will always need special care.

Women whose cesarean births have been difficult times for them can carry the emotional scars around for years, especially if they bottle up their feelings within themselves and then feel more guilt because they have them. Of course, understanding husbands, doctors, and friends can ease the problems, and gradually the negative feelings will be outweighed by the joys and trials of parenthood. But unless their emotions are ventilated, their questions are answered to their satisfaction, and the fears and burdens that have been plaguing them are understood and accepted internally, they may find them constantly resurfacing, especially during a subsequent pregnancy. When they become pregnant again is the time when most cesarean mothers find they haven't really resolved their problems about the first birth. One woman said, "I thought I had accepted having cesareans, but when I was pregnant with my second child, I would wake up every night with nightmares. The idea of having to go through that again, to have the same awful experience, was like jumping off a cliff. There was no turning back—I was heading for the cliff again."

It isn't always easy to work through the feelings, which is why the cesarean support groups that have begun to form in some areas of the country have met with such success (see page 202). They provide a forum where feelings can be shared, understood, and accepted. They supply information and the answers to the questions you may not even know you wanted to ask. Probably discovering that other people feel just the way you do is the most important help there is in freeing yourself from the entanglements a traumatic experience can engender. So, whether or not you attend meetings of an organized group, it will help to find other cesarean mothers—through your obstetrician, your hospital, your local prepared-childbirth organization— with whom you can talk and share. Some hospitals have begun to set up discussion groups for their cesarean patients, and these can be most helpful.

If your doctor is someone with whom you can freely communicate, make an appointment to talk and ask questions. Sessions with a good psychotherapist may, of course, be the answer for some people.

However you do it, get it out, work it through the best you can, so you can get on with your job of enjoying your baby. If you resolve your problems, educate yourself to the realities of this alternate method of birth, prepare, and exercise your options, you can make your next cesarean birth—if there is to be one—an experience to enjoy, a birth that is satisfying and meaningful for you and your baby.

How Other Cesarean Mothers Have Felt

"Cesarean mothers are just as concerned about their babies as other mothers are, if not more so since they seem to be making it up to their children for not 'being there' when they were born."

"I never wanted to have another baby. If it wasn't for my firm belief that a child should have a brother or a sister, I wouldn't have done it. I found out, though, that it can be much better the next time. You can prepare yourself, go to a different hospital, get a different doctor, or even try for a vaginal delivery."

"I felt so relieved by being put out of my misery after all those days of not making progress that I looked on the cesarean section as an absolute blessing."

"I've always felt my baby was delicate and sickly, even though I knew he was perfectly healthy and normal. It was because he had to be born that way. I felt like an invalid, and I guess I thought he must be, too."

"Okay, I've had a baby, but it doesn't feel like it. It feels irrelevant. What's important is how I feel."

"I was so disappointed, I felt so let down. After all our preparation and training, it happened this way."

"I felt very cheated at not being able to see the baby being born. During our Lamaze classes, our instructor went through cesareans, not in detail, but I never paid attention. Not me, it's not going to happen to me. So I did my Lamaze, but nothing was happening. The doctor said, 'I'm going to give you another hour. If you don't do something on your own, you are going to have to have a cesarean.' I don't ever remember seeing the baby. To this day, I think about the delivery obsessively."

"You don't feel right until you hold the baby in your arms. I didn't feel peace of mind until I did."

"I was livid that I was led to believe that everyone had babies the normal way."

"After all the planning, all the working, it came down to a life-and-death situation. You're glad you're alive, that the baby is alive, but there's an emotional overlay that stays with you always. You feel it's your fault, that you've failed somehow."

"My husband said it was the worst day of his life. Why is it taking so long, what are they doing, are they going to live?"

"I felt the doctor cut me off from what I wanted to do, which was to deliver this baby naturally. He didn't understand that. Even though the baby was fine, I was unhappy."

"I was asleep for my first birth and felt completely removed from the whole thing. I had depression for months. The next time, I had nine months to prepare myself. I was awake and participated in this birth. I felt this time that I had given birth. Best of all, all the old feelings of failure and depression left over from the first time were gone."

"I wish I could have felt that I took part in the whole experience. I was a bystander and my husband was completely out in the cold. I wanted to be involved instead of having such an alone feeling."

"They shouldn't mix cesareans and the others in the same room. It makes you feel so bad when you hear about their experiences, or just when you see them feeling so good and taking care of their babies. I felt I wasn't as much of a woman and a mother as they were."

"It wasn't like I'd had a baby. I had pneumonia afterward and I missed not seeing or even holding her till six days later."

"I was totally unprepared for the operation and the week that followed. If I had known more about cesareans, I think I could have been able to cope, but I knew nothing. We'd like to have another baby, but the thought of another cesarean birth terrifies me. Being in labor five days put me in a weakened condition, which accounts for some of my problems and emotional instability at the time. It's still terrifying to think about a second child."

"I felt cheated because I didn't have my husband with me, and I was confused about all that happened. I labored without medication and I did the breathing, but it didn't work out."

"*When I became pregnant with our second child, I was delighted. As the months went by, however, memories of the first experience kept surfacing like flashbacks of a nightmare. . . . Being awake the second time was a vast improvement. I felt much better afterward, too. I find the policy of not allowing you to see or hold your baby for twenty-four hours difficult to accept.*"

"*The total experience of childbirth is an emotionally painful one for me. Long before I ever became pregnant, my husband and I planned that he would help me during labor and be present at the delivery of our children when the time came. When I became pregnant, I read all the books I could find on prepared childbirth. . . . After eighteen hours of hard labor, I signed a consent form for a cesarean. The next thing I remember is waking the next morning feeling exhausted and still wondering whether or not I'd had my baby. I was disappointed, ashamed of myself, and felt somehow 'ruined.'*"

"*In retrospect, I am enraged at my doctor and the hospital because I was treated so impersonally. I did not receive my baby until thirty-six hours after the delivery. She refused to nurse and lost one and a half pounds in the first two weeks.*"

"*Although the experience was dramatic and far removed from what I had anticipated and wanted, we were relieved that both the baby and I survived a risky delivery. All in all, it was a good experience.*"

"*In a sense, I feel my baby did not come out of me, that he was given to me instead. Somehow it seems I'm not as close to him as I could have been if I touched him or saw him come out. I'm having a hard time with this.*"

"It was humiliating."

"My baby was born a year ago, but I have just this month resolved, finally, that being a cesarean mother doesn't make me biologically inferior."

"To me, breast-feeding and rooming-in helped to compensate for the loss I felt."

"The pleasure of being awake during the birth of one's baby outweighs the fear. It was wonderful seeing and touching her and feeling a part of her birth."

"I was very let down. I felt cheated because I wanted to share the experience with my husband and couldn't. I felt like an outsider during the entire birth, that I was not part of the whole experience of giving birth to my child. I am bitter about it."

"I was completely inadequate. I was sound asleep during the operation and my baby was a total little stranger when I first saw her. Once I was home, I felt inadequate all over again because I was unable to nurse after the first two weeks. I was depressed for months, maybe even a whole year."

"I felt very guilty about my 'failure' for a long time (months). The cuteness of my baby was absolutely not adequate compensation during the first days."

"I was very hopped up for one of life's beautiful experiences, and then what a letdown. I just couldn't accept what had hap-

pened to me. I couldn't feel sorry for myself because everyone kept telling me how lucky I was to have a healthy daughter. If I had had someone to talk to frankly, or even just someone to tell me I wasn't alone, I think it could have been a much better experience."

"All I felt at first was this terrible anger toward the baby. I knew that wasn't right, so I kept trying to tell myself it was crazy to feel that way. I felt it was his fault I had this pain, his fault I was in such terrible shape, and I didn't even want to see him at first. Now I'm pretty much over it. Now I'm mad at the doctor!"

"My doctor and my husband were no help at all. They both tried to make me feel better by saying things like, 'The baby is just fine, that's all that counts,' and 'Don't worry, you'll feel better in a day or so. Just relax.' I couldn't relax, and I couldn't stop thinking that I'd somehow been mutilated."

"The worst part was that I didn't feel normal. Maybe I still don't. I didn't have my baby the way I was supposed to, the way a normal woman does. I've got this scar to prove it."

"You feel all these strange ways about it but you can't tell anyone. Nobody understands because the feelings aren't rational. Who could you tell that you're sure your husband will find you repulsive now? Or that you don't think you can really love the baby? Or that you have dreams about beating up the doctor or the nurse who wouldn't come when you wanted her? I lived with all kinds of weird feelings until I found other cesarean mothers to talk to—what a relief to find out I wasn't crazy, that other women felt the same way."

"You're just not in control. Maybe anybody having an operation feels that way, I don't know, but I felt like I was no longer in charge of my life or what was happening to me. For a long time afterward, I felt completely vulnerable."

"I'd had an appendectomy a couple of years before and it was much worse than this. After the baby was born, I was up walking around the next day. I was very glad to get it over with, to be alive, and to have a healthy baby. Everyone said our baby was the best baby in the nursery."

"My first cesarean was awful and I was very upset when it happened. Though I was glad all the pain of that long labor was over, I felt my husband was cheated. He said he didn't feel that way."

"I had no desire to be awake, and my husband couldn't imagine why anybody would want to be there to see his wife opened up."

"It took me a few days to come out of the anesthesia, but, aside from that, it really wasn't bad at all. It was just something that had to happen. I accept it as that. I don't have any strange psychological feelings about having a cesarean baby."

"My doctor didn't tell me much except that he'd have to do a cesarean. That was fine with me, I wouldn't want time to think. And I had great confidence in him."

"For months I felt there was a wall between me and the baby. Nothing had gone the way we planned it, and I was obviously

very angry though I didn't realize it. I didn't expect a cesarean, I didn't want one, and I was very upset when it happened. Afterward, I didn't see the baby for six hours. He was sleeping and wouldn't open his eyes, so I just didn't feel any connection with him. Breast-feeding didn't go well and I felt like a complete failure for a long time. It wasn't until I found out that other cesarean mothers went through the same feelings that I realized I wasn't an unnatural mother."

"Naturally I was not happy I had to have a cesarean, but, given the situation, it went as well as possible. The doctor explained what he was doing and was very supportive; the nurses were great. In the operating room, a nurse described the baby to me as he was born, she brought him over to me right away, and then let my husband hold him outside until I went to the recovery room. We stayed there together for a long time and it was wonderful. It must be the hospital's policy to be concerned about your feelings because afterward the nurses made a point of being helpful and kind."

"The next thing I remember is waking up in my bed with empty arms. I could not have my baby because I was so drugged, which really depressed me because I wanted so much to hold him and feed him. Every time it was feeding time and I saw them wheel all the other babies to their mothers, I began to cry. I felt depressed, empty, in pain, and disappointed with the operation."

"The first cesarean seems to be rather awful for most of us; it was for me. But the next ones are really nothing, especially if you arrange how it's going to be done ahead of time."

❊ 15 ❊

Fathers in the
Delivery Room

To witness the birth of your own baby, to see the first moments of life, to touch and hold your newborn almost as it emerges from your body, has to be one of the most exciting events in a woman's life. And it can be one of the most exhilarating moments for your baby's father, too—if he is permitted to be present. This is true whether the birth is the usual vaginal delivery or whether the baby arrives by cesarean section using regional anesthesia. It can have a profound effect on your feelings toward each other and the baby, now and stretching far into the future.

Unfortunately, only a few cesarean fathers manage to participate in the birth experience, even though fathers of babies born in the usual way are becoming more and more accepted as part of the team in the delivery room, especially in the parts of the country where prepared childbirth has become the rule rather than the exception.

BIRTHS ARE A FAMILY AFFAIR

In many hospitals today, childbirth has been accepted as a family affair, and the father is expected to take an active part if he wants to. But not the cesarean father. After all, this birth involves surgery—husbands are not invited to watch appendectomies, are they?

There are, of course, many men who would not consider being around for the occasion. The hospital atmosphere, the surgery and blood, the fear of losing composure, all combine to keep them out in the waiting room instead of in the operating room. And there are women who do not feel a tremendous need for the presence of their partners, who feel most secure surrounded by professionals. If this is the case with you, don't feel guilty. You needn't conform to any standards or desires but your own.

The couples who are the most eager to go through a cesarean birth together are those who have prepared themselves to be partners in a vaginal delivery. They have attended classes and learned the specifics of labor and delivery. And they have faithfully practiced the breathing and relaxation techniques designed to take much of the discomfort out of the experience. The fathers have assumed the role of coach, defender, protector, participant. When they are excluded, their expectations dashed, they usually feel disappointed and cheated. Not only can they not help and take part, but they are often precipitously ejected, left behind, alone with their fears and worries. Husbands whose wives have had hurried emergency cesareans, especially, have reported they felt terrified, powerless, useless, superfluous, angry.

Often this can't be avoided. When there is a real emergency situation, there may be no time for concern for the father. But usually there is a chance for some discussion and an explanation of what is happening and why—

and very occasionally, today, a chance for the father to stay with his mate during the birth.

WHY FATHERS ARE BANNED

Whether or not a father should be allowed into the operating room has become a burning issue in several parts of the country, starting first in Boston, where groups of parents have organized to educate themselves about cesarean birth and to press for many needed changes in the traditional obstetrical routines. In any meeting of cesarean parents, the question inevitably comes up: why can't cesarean fathers be allowed at their babies' births?

The very same reasons are given for keeping fathers out of the operating room as have always been offered for barring them during an ordinary birth: "They are a source of contamination and will increase the risk of infection." "They will faint." "They will go berserk." "They will get in the way." And, peculiar to this situation, "There is something wrong with a man who wants to see his wife operated on."

The vast majority of obstetricians, and especially anesthesiologists, recoil from the idea of including the father in the room during a major abdominal operation. They believe all the usual reasons, but they have other reasons as well, not so readily told to their patients. Doctors often quite understandably find it disconcerting to attend to their work with an emotionally involved person looking over their shoulder. This is surgery, and they want to concentrate on what they are doing, and not have to make conversation and answer questions. Many are afraid the father's presence could lead to malpractice suits if anything should go wrong, or even if it merely appears that something is going wrong.

But, according to a recent study made by a group of obstetricians at the University of Michigan School of Medicine, there was no increase in the incidence of infection when fathers, gowned, masked, and scrubbed, were allowed to attend cesarean births. Nor were there any significant interferences in the surgical procedure. Not only that, but the women whose husbands were there for the delivery showed a more positive feeling toward the birth than the usual cesarean mother; they felt less lonely, less inadequate, and less helpless.

When a father is invited into the operating room, it is true he is an additional person in a crowded room, but he is stationed at his wife's head and asked not to move around. He is there, not to watch the surgery, but to share the experience as much as possible with his wife, and he normally sees no more than she does, shielded by the screen of drapes at her shoulder level.

THE REASONS TO BE THERE

Why would a man want to be present for the birth of his child when it involves surgery on the body of his wife? For the very same reasons he would want to be there for the other kind of birth: to help her, support her, reassure her, to be her friend, the person in the room who really cares about her and to whom she can turn for emotional strength; to know his baby from the moment of its arrival; to be a participant in the birth of his child, rather than an outsider who awaits word of his family from strangers. Today's young couples usually want to be together, to share experiences and work, to have fewer areas of separation between man and woman. A strong feeling of closeness usually develops between a couple in childbirth together.

An important reason for fathers to attend the births of their children is because they, too, want a close connection with their babies. Researchers Klaus and Kennell have reported that fathers who witness the birth of their children feel significantly more attached to those infants than those who don't.

Because of the pressure from groups of cesarean parents and the interest of some obstetricians, a few hospitals have begun to take down the barriers to cesarean fathers. Unfortunately, except for a few notable exceptions such as the Boston Hospital for Women, the movement has started in small hospitals that are often, to put it bluntly, looking for more business. Many of them perform relatively few deliveries, have inadequate anesthesia staffs and blood banks, and may be in danger of having to close down their obstetrical units. Sometimes they are trying to attract cesarean parents by being the first, perhaps only, hospitals in their areas to permit fathers to be present.

But, because of their example and that of the few prestigious institutions that allow it, more major hospitals have also begun to be less rigid and more understanding of the needs of their cesarean patients. It is vital that the medical centers, where most of the major trends in obstetrics are established today, start to take a lead, not only in their traditional role of improving medical and surgical techniques, but in changing standard procedures when they need changing.

WHEN IT'S APPROPRIATE FOR THE FATHER TO BE PRESENT

Most obstetricians feel there is no point in having your husband there for the cesarean birth if you are having a general anesthesia and will be sound asleep. Since his main purpose is not to watch the surgery but to share the birth experience with you, he won't be needed now for reassurance and support. There's no way he can communicate with an unconscious person. But if you are having an anesthesia that permits you to be fully conscious, then it can be appropriate to include him if you both prefer it that way. Some doctors have even begun to permit a father to witness the birth when the wife is under general anesthesia, if she wants him to be there, so that he can see and hold his baby and later relate exactly what happened during the delivery.

The cesarean birth should be an uncomplicated, non-emergency situation. In an emergency, when the baby must be delivered as quickly and expediently as possible or when there is danger of a serious problem, a father might well be in the way. This is a time when the entire medical team is under stress, and distraction cannot be tolerated. Luckily, abdominal births are seldom true emergencies, and, in fact, most are planned ahead.

If your husband wishes to accompany you into the operating room, it will be necessary to have the agreement not only of your obstetrician but also of the anesthesiologist. Unfortunately, anesthesiologists are frequently especially adamant about barring fathers or anyone else from the operating room. Perhaps it is because they have much to lose in a malpractice suit. They also have not had the opportunity to establish a meaningful doctor-patient relationship with the couple and may simply not be aware of their emotional needs.

Hospitals, too, can be impenetrable barriers to fathers. Those where cesarean babies are delivered in the regular operating rooms are usually the most rigid in their policies. When the babies are born on the obstetrical floor in delivery rooms or specially equipped cesarean rooms, the deliveries are more often regarded as the birth of a baby rather than just another surgical case. If you do find a hospital—and it may take a search—that will accept fathers, and have tracked down an obstetrician and anesthesiologist who agree, your husband will probably have to sign a form releasing the institution and the doctors from liability to him for any illness, injury, or "psychic trauma" that might follow from his presence during the birth.

Most important, if the baby's father is to be with you, he must not only wish to be there but he must be thoroughly prepared. This means he should have attended prepared-childbirth classes that included illustrated sessions on cesarean birth, and should have discussed the procedure thoroughly with the obstetrician. In other words, he should know what he is in for, just as you should. A cesarean delivery can be extremely frightening to a person who doesn't understand what is going on.

With the rise in the incidence of cesareans, some prepared-childbirth organizations have started to include more detailed classes on this alternate method of delivery, to prepare the one of every six pairs of expectant parents for whom it may become a reality. And in some communities throughout the country, separate classes have been set up for parents who know in advance that they face a cesarean birth. These and the cesarean parent support groups are just what are needed to dissipate the fears and myths and to help both parents make decisions.

Few cesarean parents today have the chance to make many decisions, including whether or not the father should be included, but each step helps to make a cesarean birth the joyful and fulfilling event it can be—the birth of a new member of the family.

Note: Since the first edition of this book was published in 1978, hospitals and obstetricians throughout the country have started to permit fathers in the delivery room, whether the delivery is vaginal or cesarean. This has come about chiefly as a result of tremendous consumer pressure, both from individual couples who search out the ideal circumstances for their birth experience and from the many cesarean support groups that have become powerful advocates of family-centered childbirth.

In some cases, another movement has been getting underway. That is to allow an appropriate substitute to accompany you into the delivery room if the baby's father isn't available. That person should be anyone who will make you feel more relaxed and comfortable during labor and delivery: your mother, another relative or close friend, or perhaps your childbirth-education instructor.

⌘ 16 ⌘

The Risks of a
Cesarean Birth

A cesarean delivery is one of the safest major operations performed today, and serious complications are extremely rare. Most of the risks of having an abdominal birth are truly minor, readily discovered, and easily treated. Because it has become so safe and offers fewer dangers than a difficult and traumatic vaginal birth, physicians seldom hesitate, in the face of complications, to make the decision to perform one.

It must be admitted, however, that any major surgery involves some risk, and a cesarean section is no exception. Just because problems do occur, even though in only a tiny number of cases, we are going to list them briefly so that you will be fully informed.

• The most obvious risk, of course, is the need for anesthesia. Going through life without surgery and without anesthesia would always be best because of very occasional allergies, accidents, and other rare problems. But the kinds of anesthesia and the procedures of administering it have improved so vastly in recent years that they offer little problem either for you or your baby.

• Wound infections after a cesarean birth occur in about one woman in every ten. The vast majority of these infections are minor and resolve by themselves or need only simple treatment. Usually, hot soaks and perhaps the addition of an antibiotic for a few days are all that is required. Sometimes, more vigorous therapy, including longer hospitalization, becomes necessary.

• Uterine infections are a fairly common occurrence after either vaginal or cesarean births, especially after multiple examinations during a long labor, prolonged rupture of the membranes, and extended use of internal fetal monitoring. The infections are usually easily managed by antibiotics, though they may prolong your stay in the hospital by a couple of days.

To prevent possible infection, your obstetrician may give you a broad-spectrum antibiotic for forty-eight hours during and immediately after your delivery. There is now firm evidence that this can significantly reduce both uterine and wound infections.

• When the bladder, normally attached to the front wall of the uterus, is moved aside in order to deliver the baby through a low-flap incision, there is the slight possibility of damage either to the bladder or to the ureters that connect it to the kidneys. Though this is a rare occurrence, it tends to happen more readily after several repeat cesarean deliveries when scarring has become extensive. If the tear is recognized and repaired during the delivery, it is of absolutely no significance. It heals and causes no further difficulty. If it goes undiscovered, however, a second operation will be needed.

• Any incision into the abdomen, particularly when it is vertical, carries with it the possibility of a hernia, which may require repair. A wound infection increases the chances of this weakening of the abdominal wall.

• A possibility of adhesions exists with every abdominal operation, though the chances are small when a low-flap incision is made.

• During the delivery of a baby by cesarean section, a large blood vessel may be inadvertently cut or torn. If this happens, multiple blood transfusions could be needed.

• Once in a great while, so rarely that most physicians never see it happen, a serious hemorrhage occurs, either because of direct injury to the uterus or because of the manner in which the placenta has implanted itself in the uterus. If the bleeding becomes uncontrollable, a hysterectomy after the baby is delivered may be the only way to solve the problem. A less drastic solution to uterine hemorrhage is tying the major blood vessels that supply the uterus—a hypogastric artery ligation.

A hysterectomy, by the way, is not an acceptable method of sterilization if the uterus is normal. If you wish to be sterilized during a cesarean birth, the preferable method is tying of the Fallopian tubes—tubal ligation.

• The chance of "one-child infertility" is heightened by a cesarean birth. Because of mild subclinical infections of the pelvic organs that may go unnoticed during the normal discomfort following the birth, tubal disease may develop and prevent another pregnancy.

• Adding to the list of improbable and rare risks is the risk of aspiration by the baby of amniotic fluid. Sometimes, because of the position of the baby, the size of the baby, or the fact that its head has become jammed into a restricted pelvis, it takes a few moments of manipulation to remove the child from the uterus. If the baby is stimulated by the physical activity or the temperature of the air to have respiratory movements, it may breathe in fluid or blood, causing a chemical kind of pneumonia that is highly irritating to the lungs and may present a risk to the baby. This is particularly serious if the surgery is being performed because of fetal distress and the baby has passed meconium (stool) into the amniotic fluid.

• And, finally, there is the small chance that a uterine scar may stretch or rupture in a subsequent pregnancy.

Many of the complications we talk about here are quite rare and, aside from minor wound or uterine infections, are truly unusual. So you shouldn't fear a cesarean birth because of the risk of a serious complication. To place it in proper perspective, losing weight, giving up smoking, and using seat belts will remove far greater risks than those associated with a cesarean delivery.

❈ 17 ❈

Choosing Your Doctor
and Hospital

As a pregnant woman and new mother, you should have excellent medical care, the most advanced equipment and techniques, sympathetic treatment, and a satisfying childbirth. Sometimes, to get all that, you must institute a search for it. Throughout this book, we have talked about the "ideal" hospital in which to have your baby delivered by cesarean section, as well as the kind of physician who will help you do the job of birthing your child. But now let's get more specific about the qualifications of hospital and doctor you should have so you may make your own checklist. Perhaps it will give you an idea of how to go about helping yourself to have a safe and dignified childbirth experience, one you will remember with pleasure the rest of your life.

CHOOSING YOUR DOCTOR

The doctor in your neighborhood to whom your friends have gone and the hospital nearest to your home may or may not be the best choices for you. Investigation is essential. When you know you are going to have a cesarean birth, your choice of obstetrician is especially important. Because it is both the birth of your baby *and* a surgical operation, you should have a very good idea just who the person is who is going to be in charge of your body and the well-being of your new infant.

Your obstetrician must be both well qualified and supportive of your needs and desires. If you live in or near a large metropolitan area, your choice of a doctor will be much easier than if you live in a more isolated community where doctors and hospitals are few.

Your first step, of course, is to gather some names of obstetricians, from friends who have had good birth experiences or from your family physician (ask which obstetrician his or her family uses). Or, even better, call the best hospital in your area and ask the Chief of Obstetrics for some recommendations. If there is a childbirth-education group and especially if there is an organization of cesarean parents, call there for names of doctors. But do not decide to go to your former obstetrician or gynecologist simply because you have used him or her before. This is not a time for the easy way out.

Once you have the names of several doctors who have been recommended by people or sources whose opinions you respect, *check their credentials.* You can phone a doctor's office and ask the nurse for information, or you can consult the *Directory of Medical Specialists* or the *American Medical Dictionary,* available in most local libraries. Find out where and when they did their residencies and make sure they are *diplomates* of the American Board of Obstetrics and Gynecology.

If a doctor is not listed among the board-certified obstetricians in your city and state, that means he/she has not taken or passed the specialty board examinations. Any M.D. can legally deliver a baby, just as any of them can perform brain surgery, but not all of them are qualified to do a good job, especially when there may be complications. Passing the specialty boards—becoming a diplomate—is the very least qualification you must look for in your obstetrician.

A listing as a *fellow* of the American College of Obstetrics and Gynecology is not the same as a diplomate and does not mean this doctor has passed the boards. Nor does membership in local, state, or national medical societies. Any M.D. can join a medical society simply by paying dues.

It is reasonable to assume that an obstetrician who is on the teaching staff of a medical school and works out of a teaching institution will be a good choice for you, simply because a teaching appointment carries with it implications of expertise and knowledge of the most modern obstetrical information, techniques, and philosophies. It is not always true, of course, but a faculty appointment almost forces a physician to maintain an overall high level of medical practice. So, if you live within some miles of a teaching hospital, it would be wise to ask there first for a recommendation.

Among your other considerations in choosing your obstetrician is whether it is important to you that you have a one-to-one relationship with that person. Many physicians today have group practices, with perhaps three, four, or five doctors working together. The groups often offer superior medical care, but it may be disturbing to you not to know just which one of the group is going to deliver your baby. And if you have a particular need for a physician who shares your philosophy about childbirth methods, it may not be easy to find a group of doctors who all have the same approach. You must decide if this is of serious concern to you, and talk to all of them if need be.

If you wish to have your baby in a hospital that offers a specific kind of care, then you will have to choose a doctor who is privileged to deliver babies in that hospital. Some women choose a certain hospital because that institution is known to be the most technologically advanced or medically sophisticated in the area; others choose a hospital because it offers them more control over their own childbirths—choice of anesthesia, for example; a rooming-in plan; liberal visiting privileges for fathers or even fathers in the delivery room. If you know you want to deliver in a certain hospital, call the obstetrical department and ask for the names of doctors affiliated with the institution.

IF YOU WANT A VAGINAL DELIVERY

When you would like to attempt a vaginal delivery after having had a previous cesarean birth, finding the right doctor becomes even more difficult. Most obstetricians believe that "once a cesarean, always a cesarean" is safest and wisest for every woman. They feel it is much less risky, and would not want to take the chance that it might not work out.

Nevertheless, a vaginal delivery may be a possibility for your next birth, depending, of course, on many medical realities (see Chapter 3). To find an obstetrician who is even willing to discuss the possibility of a vaginal delivery may not be easy. You will have to call many hospitals for recommendations, perhaps travel miles from home to find both the appropriate person and hospital. The physician who delivers you vaginally after a previous cesarean birth must not only have had experience doing it, and privileges in a hospital with twenty-four hour anesthesia, laboratory, and blood-bank coverage, but he (she) must be willing to spend many hours in the hospital while you labor. His constant presence is essential, and many physicians simply do not have the time or the inclination for it.

INTERVIEWING YOUR CANDIDATES

Now, armed with the names of one or more qualified obstetricians, you are ready for the next step—personal interviews or consultations with them to find out if their practices, views, and philosophies about childbirth match yours. If you are a woman who prefers an obstetrician who will take over and assume full responsibility, your choice will be much easier than if you are seeking to play a larger part in your own childbirth.

Most women, especially when they know they are destined for a cesarean birth, are more concerned with the professional ability of their obstetrician than with his or her philosophy. But the person who shares this important, intimate, and exciting event in your life should be someone whom you like and respect, someone with whom you will feel secure enough to reveal yourself comfortably both physically and emotionally.

If you are among the growing number of women who actively prepare and educate themselves for childbirth, either vaginal or cesarean, your choice may be especially important to you, because one of your major concerns will be to find an obstetrician who believes in sharing the childbirth, at least to some extent, with his or her patients.

SETTING UP THE MEETING

Call the doctor's office and explain in a pleasant, nondefiant manner that you would like an appointment with the doctor just to talk. If you plan to meet with the doctor together with your husband, let this be known. Remember that this is going to be a close relationship for many months, culminating in the birth of your baby, and you have a right to meet the person who may be working so closely with you during a very important time in your life.

If it is easier for you to handle, make an appointment for your first prenatal visit, and combine this with your inquiries. But don't be afraid to ask the questions you'd planned to ask.

Don't be surprised if your request for an interview is met with some hostility. After all, most of us are not used to having our practices, ideas, and philosophies questioned, though it's time they were. If the hostility is powerful, cross that name off your list, and go on to the next. But don't be put off by the assistant or nurse who answers the telephone; if she is resistant, ask to speak to the doctor. As the consumer movement grows, more and more physicians are learning that the interview is becoming expected. Some will charge for the visit, but many do not. Even if you must pay for the consultation, it can be a worthwhile investment.

Take note, when you reach the physician's office, whether you are kept waiting for an unreasonable length of time. It won't be pleasant or convenient to have to wait for an hour or more each time you have a prenatal examination. Make conversation with the nurse or receptionist; sometimes you can make some judgments about the doctor by the people he (she) hires to deal with patients.

Once you are in the doctor's office, sitting down and talking, ask questions about all the matters that especially concern you, and let him (or her) know your own desires for your delivery. If you are not sure you are going to require a cesarean, perhaps you will want to know his attitudes about prepared childbirth if this is what you would prefer. In any case, his attitudes will clue you in to the way he works. Ask whether he recommends that his patients go to classes and whether there are any in the area specifically for cesarean parents.

Discuss the kinds of drugs and anesthesia he (she) would use for a cesarean delivery and his feelings about allowing you to be conscious and awake for the birth if you would like to be. Ask if he objects to fathers in the operating room; whether they may come to prenatal visits; if you may hold your baby in the delivery room; how soon you can breast-feed. Inquire how long the baby will be separated from you; how quickly you will be able to get out of bed.

If rooming-in is important to you, discuss his feelings about it. Find out if he is enthusiastic about breast-feeding if that's what you plan to do. Ask what he charges for a cesarean delivery and what your other costs would be. Find out which ones are covered by your medical insurance plan.

When you get the answers, you are going to have to sort them out. Doctors who are decisively one way or another are easy to figure. But sometimes you will get replies that will require your own interpretation as to both meaning and sincerity.

If you go into the office looking for an argument or presenting your views in a rigid, defiant manner, you can be pretty sure the doctor, whose time may be short, would just as soon you'd go elsewhere, no matter what his obstetrical and human philosophy is. So if you want an honest discussion, don't go there prepared for a confrontation.

MAKING AN EVALUATION

Let's assume the doctor gives you the answers you are looking for. Do you feel comfortable with him (her)? Can you talk to him easily? Does he seem straightforward, answer your questions fully, and give you enough time? Does he treat you as an equal, an intelligent human being who can understand words of more than two syllables and can comprehend most medical and anatomical terms? Is he respectful? In other words, do you like him? Is he someone you will want to be involved with so intimately? Be careful not to judge solely on personality, however—when it comes to a choice, medical excellence must come first. Ideally, you will find a doctor who will combine all or most of the qualities that are important to you.

If you decide this is not, or may not be, the person for you, go on to the next one on your list. Many women today talk to four or five obstetricians before settling on one.

When you live in a small community far from a metropolitan area and do not wish to travel to find the ideal doctor for you, you may have to make compromises because there is a limited number of obstetricians available to you. Choose the person who most closely meets your needs and then try to educate him throughout your pregnancy as to what it is you want from this childbirth. If, even in midpregnancy, you decide that you have made a poor choice of doctors, don't hesitate to change. It's best to change early, but it's better to change late than to continue on with someone with whom you know you will not have a good experience.

Don't hesitate to talk to your doctor about your feelings and wishes, even if he seems resistant to ideas different from his own. You are the consumer, you are paying for this person's services, and you have a right to the kind of care you want. That doesn't mean you'll get it, but if enough women begin to realize their "pregnant power," changes are going to continue to be made.

So many more women are choosing doctors more carefully today, pressuring them to alter some of their sacred traditional methods, speaking out for what they want, and asking for more dignified treatment, that even the most conservative physicians have begun to reexamine themselves, their attitudes, and the way they work. We are all changing, and that is good.

CHOOSING YOUR HOSPITAL

There are multitudes of hospitals in this country that should not be allowed to provide obstetrical services simply because they cannot do a good job. They are not well enough equipped, they do too few deliveries to keep up with the newest techniques, and they do not have a staff complete or competent enough to provide safe care.

If, at the last moment, a cesarean delivery becomes necessary, these hospitals are unprepared. An anesthesiologist must be called in from perhaps an hour away, an operating-room nurse must be rounded up, laboratory and X-ray technicians may never be found in time, the blood bank may be closed or nonexistent, and a pediatric intensive-care unit may never have been contemplated or even vaguely approximated.

In an emergency, when a baby must be delivered quickly in order to survive in good health, a delay of forty-five minutes or an hour may be much too long. If that is what your hospital will require to get ready for a cesarean delivery, you are not in the best hands.

A planned cesarean birth, one that is scheduled to occur before the onset of labor, does allow plenty of time for all the necessary ingredients of a safe birth to be assembled. But a vaginal delivery after a previous cesarean birth must *never* take place in a hospital that is not constantly prepared for immediate emergency surgery.

If you live in an area within reasonable distance from a fully equipped hospital, it would therefore be wise to choose that hospital. Even with a repeat cesarean birth planned to occur just before term, you will want to make sure your baby is mature enough to get along nicely in the outside world. Are the necessary laboratory tests available in your hospital or at a nearby facility?

The very best hospitals, from a medical point of view, are those with twenty-four-hour anesthesia coverage (this means the constant presence and readiness of trained anesthesiologists or anesthetists), a full-time blood bank (staffed around the clock so that blood is always ready within minutes in case it is needed), a total operating-room staff available at all times, plus adequate means of labor monitoring. Most major hospitals have all of these facilities.

These are probably the most important considerations in choosing a hospital in which to have a baby. Unfortunately, the large medical centers with the best facilities are usually the hospitals with the most inflexible policies. And some of the small, ill-equipped, understaffed institutions have become the most amenable to change because they are seeking more obstetrical business.

But there is a trend today toward smaller, more intimate hospitals providing competent medical care, as well as a trend in larger hospitals toward flexibility and a more homelike pleasant atmosphere in which to give birth. The only way you, as the consumer, can find out which hospital in your area best fills both needs is to investigate them.

THE HUMAN ELEMENT

The second most important consideration in choosing the hospital best for you is the prevailing attitude of the place. This is demonstrated by hospital "policies," both written and unwritten, and by the personnel.

Check with your obstetrician and/or with the hospital about its anesthesiologists. If you wish to be awake for the birth, is there an anesthesiologist who can and will give you conduction anesthesia? Is there someone who is trained to give epidurals? Does the hospital have a rooming-in plan, and does (or can) it apply to cesarean mothers who want it? Are fathers allowed in the labor room, the delivery room? If not, how and when are they informed about what is happening? How long must your baby, assuming it is healthy, remain in the nursery before it can be brought to you? Can you arrange to breast-feed the first day? Is the nursing staff cooperative with breast-feeding cesarean mothers? Are there open visiting hours for fathers?

Are there sufficient nurses on the obstetrical floor? Have they the reputation for being pleasant and helpful? This is most important to know, since a major complaint of cesarean mothers is the often poor treatment they receive from hospital personnel.

Many hospitals now permit daily visits by the new baby's brothers and sisters. Some provide a visiting room and others allow sibling visitation in private rooms. You're going to be in the hospital longer than other mothers. If it's important to you to see your children, find out if the hospital allows it. Obviously, the small visitors should be free from the common infectious childhood diseases.

MAKING THE DECISION

If you can find a hospital that combines excellent facilities *and* a compassionate human approach toward its childbearing patients, you are not only extremely lucky but also very rare. More likely, you will probably have to make some compromises, depending on your priorities. You may wish to choose a smaller hospital that does not have every facility and capability we have discussed, because a pleasant experience is more important to you. Or you may decide to opt for a hospital that emphasizes prepared childbirth and relaxed rules. The important thing is to keep your choices in mind.

MAKE YOUR DOCTOR YOUR ADVOCATE

When you must choose a hospital with rigid policies, you may be able to use your obstetrician as your personal advocate. If he (she) is willing to go along with some of your requests—allowing your husband in the operating room, getting your baby soon after the delivery, breast-feeding the first day if that is possible, for example—perhaps he will speak out in your behalf. Hospitals rarely change their routines on their own, but may respond to requests from their doctors and pressure from their patients. If your doctor is on your side, your chances are good that some changes may be made. Remind him that you would like your cesarean delivery to be a fulfilling child-birth experience and not merely a surgical procedure.

THE COSTS OF A CESAREAN BIRTH

Having a baby today is never cheap, no matter how you do it, but having one by cesarean delivery can put an awful strain on the family pocketbook, especially when it is unexpected. Medical insurance plans do pay higher benefits for cesarean sections, however, and may offset some of your expenses.

It is general practice in this country for physicians to charge more for cesarean section deliveries, even though the operation may be a simple one and take much less of the doctor's time than the usual delivery. The obstetrical fee, which covers prenatal care, the delivery, postoperative care, and several postnatal visits, could cost, in the New York metropolitan area, between $800 and $1,200. Elsewhere, the fees are usually less.

Then there is the anesthesiologist, who must be paid; in New York, this fee will probably come to between $150 and $250. A private pediatrician who examines the newborn baby will charge $50 to $100, assuming the baby is healthy and does not require any extraordinary medical care. If it does, your costs will skyrocket from there.

The hospital bill for the average hospital stay for mother and baby may come to another $2,500, again assuming there are no unusual complications requiring intensive medical care for the infant or for you.

The cost of medical care is so extraordinary in New York and several other large cities that few insurance plans will pay the total surgical and medical charges. In other parts of the country, however, some physicians will accept the fees paid by the medical insurance plans as payment in full for their services.

Before too many years pass, some kind of federal medical assistance will surely be enacted to provide comprehensive maternity benefits to all women in the country. In the meantime, you should be sure to discuss the costs with your doctor in a preliminary interview or early in your pregnancy. If the charges seem out of line, you may wish to make the cost a part of your considerations in making a choice. Hospital costs vary, too, both from one part of the country to another and within a community. Find out what they are before making your decision.

⊠ 18 ⊠

Your Rights as a Pregnant
Patient and New Mother

Your obstetrician is not likely to ask your opinion about
whether or not to perform an unplanned cesarean section.
This is a critical medical decision, and you will have to be
guided by his/her judgment. Few women are well enough
informed about obstetrics to argue the merits of their own
case in the face of an emergency.

However, there are some rights and privileges that are
reasonable to expect when you have a cesarean birth, and
we are going to list some of them to give you an idea of
what to look for, ask for, or perhaps insist upon. Many of
these rights are listed in "The Pregnant Patient's Bill of
Rights." *

YOUR RIGHT TO KNOW WHAT
IS HAPPENING

Sometimes when a cesarean birth is unexpected and is
performed because of a sudden and serious medical crisis,

* You may obtain a copy by sending a stamped self-addressed envelope to the
Committee on Patients' Rights, Box 1900, New York, N.Y. 10001.

there will not be time for the physician to explain what is going on. If your life or your baby's life is at stake, the main concern is for survival and your emotional concerns must be pushed aside. The only thing that matters at that moment is a quick and safe delivery of the baby.

But, in most cases, even an "emergency" cesarean birth is not performed immediately, and there is time for a concise explanation of the situation. When there is time for an explanation, you should have one, in whatever detail you wish. In other words, you have the right to raise your hand and say, in essence, "Wait a minute. Remember me? I am the person to whom this is happening. Tell me what you are doing to me and why you are doing it."

The answers you will get will depend on the personality of the doctor you have chosen as your obstetrician—some physicians will resist sharing their medical decision-making with you and will try to put you off with "We're doing it to save your baby." Not good enough. Even if you must wait until after the delivery for the kind of information you are seeking, it is important to know. It is your right to ask questions and to get answers.

YOUR RIGHT TO KNOW WHAT ANESTHESIA YOU WILL RECEIVE

If there is time, and if the available anesthesiologist has the capability of giving you the kind of anesthesia you choose—general, which will put you to sleep, or conduction, which will allow you to be conscious for the delivery—then you should have the choice. In a real emergency, you will probably get whatever anesthesia is quickest, easiest, and safest to administer in that hospital. Sometimes every kind of anesthesia is not available to you, nor is it always appropriate. But you may inquire, and your preference should certainly be considered.

If your cesarean birth is planned ahead, you will surely

have a chance to discuss, and perhaps choose, your anesthesia, and an opportunity to meet and talk with the anesthesiologist. Ask to see this person in plenty of time before the delivery—it will make you feel much more secure and confident to have formed at least a minimal relationship with someone who is going to play an important part in your life.

Your Right to Know What Other Drugs You Will Receive

If you have a cesarean section unexpectedly after laboring for some hours, you may already have received some drugs for pain or apprehension. Usually, however, these drugs are kept to a minimum, since it is known that they cross the placenta to the baby. Also, if you have trained for prepared childbirth, you may not have needed much medication.

Once you know you are having a cesarean delivery, you have the right to ask the doctor not to give you any preoperative medications—analgesias, tranquilizers, or sedatives—if you plan to be awake for the delivery. Go on record that you do not want them. In some hospitals, the drugs are routinely added to the intravenous solution and all you will know is that you were drowsy during the birth when you wanted to be alert.

Again, *if* you are going to be awake, you may ask your doctor not to give you any pain medication during or immediately after the delivery unless you request it. Sometimes, medication or more anesthesia is given toward the end of the delivery or the repair as a way to relieve discomfort or potential anxiety. If you have planned to see your baby in the delivery room and perhaps hold it in the recovery room, you won't want to be knocked out. In any case, conduction anesthesia is usually effective for at least a half hour after the delivery is completed.

YOUR RIGHT TO ASK FOR CERTAIN TESTS

When you are having a planned cesarean birth that is scheduled to occur before you go into labor, you should make certain that the proper maturity tests are made. Unless there is a reason why the baby must be delivered *now*—and that means it is in jeopardy if it remains in the uterus any longer—there is no excuse for having a premature baby by cesarean section. There are ways available today to test fetal maturity (see Chapter 5).

YOUR RIGHT TO HAVE YOUR BABY WITH YOU AFTER BIRTH

Because it is so important to the mother-infant relationship to spend time with your new baby immediately after its birth (see Chapter 11), you have the right to ask if this can be arranged. Traditional hospital routines separate mother and baby, especially after a cesarean birth, but the trend today is to eliminate that separation as much as possible when the baby is healthy—as it almost always is.

Speak to your obstetrician *before* the delivery, if you can, to see if it would be possible to have your baby brought to you in the recovery room if you are having conduction anesthesia, and to find out how soon after you are back in your room you will have the baby. Let it be known that, as soon as you feel well enough, you will want your baby. Certainly, twelve hours after delivery is the very most a normal healthy infant must be kept under observation, and even that long is very rarely necessary.

YOUR RIGHT TO BREAST-FEED

It has always been assumed that cesarean mothers are not going to breast-feed their babies; that, because of their postoperative discomfort, they will want the job of feeding taken over by the hospital staff. In recent years, however, more new mothers are intent on breast-feeding, and more cesarean mothers are deciding not to be put off from this important function by their abdominal incisions. Cesarean mothers can breast-feed as well as any other mother, though they may have a little more trouble getting going initially. This is not because of the method of delivery—a cesarean section does not affect the production of milk—but because they may be separated from their babies longer than women who delivered vaginally and because they may be quite uncomfortable for the first couple of days.

Do you want to breast-feed? Tell your obstetrician before the delivery, and again after the delivery. Enlist the aid of your pediatrician, if necessary, to get your baby early enough for easy feeding, and have your husband act as advocate and helper. Ask that your baby not be fed formula in the nursery, and that he or she be brought to you on a three-hour schedule for feeding (see Chapter 12).

YOUR RIGHT TO DIGNIFIED CHILDBIRTH AND CARE

If you ever feel—before, during, or after the birth—that you are not being treated with respect and caring, that your own special needs, emotionally and physically, are being ignored or treated shabbily, you have the right to complain and to ask for changes. Look for help from your obstetrician, the nurses, the head nurse, the hospital administrator, your pediatrician, your husband, or other members of your family. You will be able to effect changes immediately for your own benefit, and your voice will be added to many others that are helping to bring about more humanized and dignified childbirth in this country. When you are home again, write letters to the hospital if you have constructive suggestions to make, ideas that could make its handling of childbirth better. Cesarean mothers are only now becoming vocal in their search for a happy birth experience.

⊠ 19 ⊠

Cesarean Prevention

With a phenomenally high cesarean birth rate in the United States, every woman who is about to have a baby takes a chance that she, too, will have an abdominal delivery. When it's necessary, a cesarean obviously provides a birth route that saves mothers and babies from traumatic or damaging difficulties. But a major abdominal operation always involves an element of risk as well as postoperative discomfort and a prolonged recovery period, besides being a psychological problem for some women. Therefore, reducing the number of cesareans has become a subject of intense interest among doctors, medical institutions, groups of concerned citizens, and governmental and professional agencies.

The consensus is that many cesareans can be safely avoided.

Let's talk about some of the ways you and your doctor may manage to avoid a cesarean, this time or the next time around.

Vaginal Birth After a Previous Cesarean (VBAC)

The most effective way of preventing a surgical delivery is to forsake the old rule "Once a cesarean, always a cesarean," which we discussed in Chapter 3. The largest single reason for a cesarean delivery is a *previous* cesarean delivery. About 99 percent of all women who have had this kind of birth once have them again for their next babies, and at least a third of the cesareans in American hospitals are performed for this reason alone.

The truth is that at least half—and probably many more—of the women who have already had cesareans can safely deliver their subsequent babies in the traditional way—through the birth canal. The first surgery may have been performed for a reason that no longer exists: toxemia, or a breech presentation, for example, or disproportion between your pelvis and the size of the baby. Perhaps the primary cesarean was simply a precaution, a response to an indication that maybe something was amiss. But, whatever the cause of your first, or second, or third cesarean, you should be reevaluated this time around to decide if another is really necessary. In the last few years, obstetricians in many respected major medical institutions have made it a policy to encourage their patients who meet certain criteria to have a "trial of labor" to try to accomplish a vaginal delivery before resorting to more surgery.

So, if you don't want an automatic "repeat," tell your obstetrician you want to try for a vaginal birth this time. Or, if you haven't already chosen your physician, look for one who is willing to give you every opportunity to avoid the surgical route. Remember that it's essential that the hospital has an around-the-clock anesthesiologist on the premises as well as all the other support systems detailed in Chapter 3, just in case you require another cesarean after all.

AVOIDING A BIG WEIGHT GAIN

If you start out your pregnancy vastly overweight, or if you gain more than about forty pounds during the nine months, you have increased your chances of requiring a cesarean delivery. That's because you are much more likely to have an oversize baby (over eight and one-half pounds) who may have a hard time making it through your pelvic passageway.

It's never wise to restrict your nutritional intake too much during your pregnancy, and it's very important that you eat sufficient calories in a completely balanced diet the entire nine months so that the baby, the placenta, and the uterus are strong and healthy. So, if you are overweight, try to lose the excess weight *before* you conceive; don't go on a diet after you are pregnant because you risk providing insufficient nourishment for the baby. But don't go overboard either, using your pregnancy as an excuse to gain large amounts of weight. Try to keep your gain between twenty and twenty-five pounds.

TAKING ADVANTAGE OF GRAVITY

The most common medical indication for a cesarean delivery of first babies is "failure to progress in labor" (uterine inertia). Your obstetrician must make a decision when your labor lasts for many hours without sufficient dilatation of the cervix or descent of the baby's head into the pelvis: should the labor be allowed to continue longer or is a cesarean the answer?

When a woman enters the hospital in early labor, the usual procedure in this country today is to put her right into bed. There she stays, flat on her back, often hooked up to a fetal heart monitor and with an IV in her arm, confined in one position until she delivers the baby one way or another.

But there is an encouraging trend back to an old idea: allowing a woman in the early stages of labor to sit up, get out of bed, walk around the room, pace up and down the hall, and, in fact, do almost anything she feels like doing while she waits for her baby to be born. Sitting, standing, and squatting allow the force of gravity to help the fetus drop down into the pelvis, effacing and dilating the cervix in preparation for birth. It also takes pressure off the vena cava (the major blood vessel of the uterus), permitting a better blood flow to the fetus. Obviously, if moving around helps the labor to progress normally, it diminishes the risk of a cesarean.

One common objection to this trend is that it's impossible for a laboring woman to get out of bed and walk around if she is attached by wires to a fetal heart monitor. Though monitors are often unnecessary and have been accused of promoting more cesareans, they have also proved essential in many instances as the best way to get good information about the condition of the baby inside the uterus.

Some hospitals are already using a new kind of monitor that uses radio signals instead of wires to transmit its reports about your uterine contractions and the baby's heartbeat, so you can be tracked wherever you are. But, even if you must be attached by wires to the monitor, there is seldom a need for a constant and continuous readout. Intermittent readings are usually sufficient. When you first arrive at the labor room, you may be monitored in bed for about half an hour. Then every thirty minutes or so after that you can stop your ambulations and lie down again for five or ten minutes of abdominal monitoring. Except in rare instances, this is enough, and if the movement and gravity help your labor to progress more rapidly, you have diminished your chances of having a cesarean.

The birthing chair also works on the gravity principle. Because it allows you to sit up, it makes pushing (the second stage of labor) more effective. But almost the same results can be achieved by sitting up in bed or in a chair until the baby's head is about to come out.

NOURISHMENT DURING EARLY LABOR

Women are rarely permitted to eat or drink during labor because there is a chance that they may eventually require a general anesthesia if they must have a cesarean; but quite clearly, the woman in labor needs both fluid replacement and calories to continue such strenuous physical exertion for any length of time. Some doctors are now permitting their patients to drink liquids and eat easily digestible foods in early labor. If the labor is prolonged, fluids, calories, and electrolytes may be readily replaced intraveneously.

AVOIDING EXCESSIVE MEDICATION

Another way to help keep your labor moving along at optimum speed is to take as little medication as possible, especially in the early stages. Because it is a documented fact that narcotics and tranquilizers can interfere with the labor process, slowing or sometimes even stopping the contractions, this is another excellent reason to take a childbirth-education class so you can help yourself manage with a minimum of drugs.

The more relaxed and free of tension you are, the less discomfort you will feel. To an amazing degree, pain is a matter of personal interpretation and a summary of both internal and external circumstances. Without fear, you may experience it as more uncomfortable than painful. In any case, you can always cope with pain and pressure more easily when you know what is going on and feel in control. You can work *with* your contractions, not against them, and this helps the uterus to relax and the cervix to dilate more readily. Studies have shown that mothers who actively participate in their childbirth tend to have significantly shorter labors and need smaller amounts of medication.

If your baby's father can be with you—well-trained and motivated—he can provide both assistance and security. If he isn't available, you may want to ask someone else with whom you feel close to be with you and coach you in the labor room—a relative, a friend, or perhaps your childbirth-education instructor. Even if the father is present, you may still want a childbirth coach with you to help you cope effectively with labor.

AVOIDING EPIDURAL ANESTHESIA IN LABOR

Epidural anesthesia that numbs your lower body has become quite common for women who don't want to contend with labor pains. It does make labor a breeze, but it may well increase your chances of requiring a cesarean delivery. The drug often interferes with the patterns of normal labor, sometimes slowing the contractions down to the point where you require yet another drug, oxytocin, to stimulate them artificially. In addition, it may also blunt your reflex urge to push during the second stage of labor when your active help is needed.

RETHINKING THE ELECTIVE INDUCTION OF LABOR

Except in unusual circumstances, it is a bad idea to have an elective induction of labor, to schedule your baby's arrival simply for your or your doctor's convenience. Elective inductions are one way to start down the path toward a cesarean delivery because it is not always possible to predict exactly when your baby will be ready to be born. If the induction is done too early, your cervix may never dilate sufficiently to permit a vaginal delivery and, besides, your baby may be premature.

Occasionally, there are valid medical reasons for the obstetrician to decide to use a drug to induce labor. Perhaps you are several weeks overdue and the fetus is very large, or you have a health problem that causes concern for the baby's welfare inside your body. Even so, it's wise to get a second opinion on the need for induction before agreeing to it. Because failed inductions are a common cause for cesareans, it should be carefully determined that the procedure is really needed and that the baby is ready.

Even if your membranes have already broken, an induction can be held off quite safely for twenty-four to forty-eight hours if careful monitoring of maternal and fetal pulse and white blood count show no indication of infection. About 90 percent of women begin labor spontaneously within that number of hours after the waters break. If there is no infection and time is allowed to pass, it's doubtful that you will require a drug to start your contractions.

REEVALUATING THE SIGNS OF "FETAL DISTRESS"

Since so many cesareans are performed because the fetus is perceived to be in some difficulty inside the uterus and it's decided it would be better off delivered, it makes excellent sense to be quite sure the difficulty is real. Current thinking is that a cesarean should not be performed because of "fetal distress" until that is quite obviously the case—confirmed by fetal blood studies. The fetal heart can slow temporarily for many reasons, the vast majority of them quite harmless. Only when there is a decreased oxygen supply to the baby is there usually a need for concern. Most large hospitals today have the facilities on hand for measuring the pH (alkalinity/acidity) of the fetal blood, along with its content of oxygen and carbon dioxide, so that fetal distress is taken out of the realm of guesswork and becomes a much more scientific decision.

An additional way to be more certain that the distress is real and requires emergency action is to be checked out by a hand-held fetoscope and a second fetal monitor. Monitors have been known to malfunction.

TURNING THE BABY AROUND

Many cesarean deliveries of first babies occur because these infants decide not to come into the world headfirst. Instead, they arrive as breeches. Though breech babies—especially frank breeches who present their buttocks first and weigh between five and one-half to eight pounds—may be safely delivered vaginally by obstetricians with experience, there is no question that the use of cesareans in such cases has been responsible for a significant drop in damaged children. So most breeches will continue to be born surgically.

But why not try to turn the baby around? Using an old technique called "external version" in the last month of pregnancy, it's quite possible to convert a breech position into a vertex (headfirst).

External version is accomplished by the obstetrician who very carefully manipulates the fetus, pushing and pulling it into the proper position by pressing on the abdominal wall with his (her) hands. At the same time, a real-time sonographic scanner is used to keep a close watch on the fetal position as well as the fetal heart rate. There is a small risk of initiating labor, and occasionally the maneuver won't work at all or the baby turns around again. But there's no harm done and, if the baby is coaxed into coming out headfirst, one more cesarean delivery has been prevented.

To help yourself turn the baby around, there are a few other methods thought by some people to induce the fetus to reverse its position, though there are no scientific studies that prove it, merely testimony. One is to spend twenty minutes or so on your hands and knees a few times a day. Another: on a slant board or ironing board propped against a piece of furniture at a 45-degree angle, lie down with your head toward the floor. Remain in this position for about twenty minutes. Repeat three or four times a day.

We have no way of knowing whether these techniques

work, but if you can manage to remain on your hands and knees, or lying head down on a slant board for that much time each day, you won't do yourself any harm—and who knows, you may accomplish your goal.

Obviously, the attitude of your obstetrician to these issues, as well as his (her) adherence to rigid obstetrical "rules" such as a specific limitation on the length of the second stage of labor (the pushing stage), will have a lot to do with your ultimate chances of having a cesarean.

Sources of Information

For further information about classes or support groups for cesarean parents, write to:

Nationwide and International
The International Childbirth
  Education Association,
  Inc. (ICEA)
P.O. Box 20048
Minneapolis, MN 55420

Cesarean Prevention
  Movement
1008 Westcott Street
Syracuse, NY 13210

American Society of
  Psycho-Prophylaxis in
  Obstetrics (ASPO)
1411 K Street, N.W.
Washington, DC 20005

La Leche League
  International
9616 Minneapolis Avenue
Franklin Park, IL 60131

Cesarean Birth Association
125 North 12th Street
New Hyde Park, NY 11040

Arizona
The Cesarean Birth Group,
  Ltd.
11011 North 45th Lane
Glendale 85304

California
C/Birth, Inc.
P.O. Box 5512
Orange 92667

Cesarean Birth Council
  International
P.O. Box 6081
San Jose 95150

Connecticut
Cesarean Parents' Group
617 West Main Street
Amston 06231

Florida
Council for Cesarean
  Awareness
5520 S.W. 92nd Avenue
Miami 33165

Illinois
C-Section of Northern
  Illinois
1220 Gentry
Hoffman Estates 60195

Indiana
Cesarean Association for
  Resources and Education
9020 Rosewood Lane
Indianapolis 46240

Maryland
Maryland Cesarean Section
  Association
P.O. Box 10431
Baltimore 21209

Massachusetts
C/SEC Inc.
22 Forest Road
Framingham 01701

Michigan
Cesarean Childbirth Concern
4333 Wagon Wheel
Lansing 48717

New York
Cesarean Parents Committee
Westchester ASPO
Box 125 Scarborough
Briarcliff Manor 10510

Pennsylvania
Cesarean Parents of Scranton
R.D. #5, Box 177
Clarks Summit 18411

Texas
Cesarean Awareness of Dallas
1722 Leicester Street
Garland 75042

Wisconsin
Cesarean Parents
5636 West Burleigh Street
Milwaukee 53210

Index